THE
VINTAGE
YEARS

ALSO BY FRANCINE TODER

When Your Child is Gone: Learning to Live Again

Your Kids Are Grown: Moving on With and Without Them

The Vintage Years

Finding Your Inner Artist
(Writer, Musician, Visual Artist)
After Sixty

Francine Toder, Ph.D.

Aziri Books
Palo Alto, California

Aziri Books

2085 East Bayshore Road, # 50398
Palo Alto, California 94303

Printed in the United States of America

First Edition, 2013

Library of Congress Control Number: 2012949911

Toder, Francine

The Vintage Years: Finding Your Inner Artist (Writer, Musician, Visual Artist) After Sixty / by Francine Toder — 1st ed.

Includes bibliographic references and index.

ISBN: 978-0-9882059-2-5 (hardcover: alk. paper)

Aging—Psychological and cognitive aspects; creativity

Lifestyle—Fine arts

Health & Wellness

AziriBooks.com

To Yvette—dear aunt, more like a loving and wise big sister, who embodies and expresses the essence of late-blooming artistry.

Contents

Mort: mixed media, large installations

Introduction

Kathleen: poet and non-fiction writer

Stan: fiction writer

Michelle: novelist

Anne: haiku and local history writer

Caroline: historical memoirist

Yvette: poet and short story writer

Bette: writer and sketch artist

Part III

Wisdom and the Brain

Wisdom and Evolutionary Psychology

Wisdom and Aging Artists from the Past

Wisdom, Exercise, and the Brain: Creating Synergy

Sealing the Wisdom: Summing-up and Encore

Retirement: Rule in or Rule Out

Retirement Decision Tree # 1

The Influence of Personal Style

Consider the Possibilities

The Working Artist

Resources and Opportunities

Decision Tree 2

Different Strokes for Different Folks

Preface

I didn't set out to write a book that evolved into *The Vintage Years*. I began by pondering, as psychologists do, my current life stage at sixty-plus chronological years, referred to variously as late adulthood, the senior years, the golden days, or less affectionately as old age or over the hill.

Change is inevitable. Time passes swiftly. I look back at the circuitous path of my more than forty-year career as a psychologist—first on a college campus, later in private practice—and the many serendipitous twists and turns that led me to writing this book. Perhaps it was simply a matter of shifting priorities or interests, but as I approached age seventy, I began to feel wanderlust for exploring what could yet be discovered in my own life.

"What's next?" and "If not now, when?" surfaced as nagging questions begging for answers. These could be the quintessential questions of what I call the Vintage Years—the first stage in life without a clearly laid-out path and set of expectations. At this point in our lives, many of us are still physically active, intellectually curious, emotionally stable, and yearning for meaningful ways to spend our time. But how?

Trying to practice what I preach and personally searching for ways to experience more pleasure and new meaning, I wondered how to satisfy my wish to explore and discover. It didn't take long to embark on what will hopefully become a project for the rest of my life.

Rather impulsively, and most probably because of my association with a chamber music institute that infuses my community with astonishingly beautiful music each summer, I went to look at cellos in a San Francisco shop that sells and rents stringed instruments. Knowing nothing more about the cello than the smooth and mellow music it can produce, I rented one along with a case to transport and protect it. In rapid succession, I bought a self-instruction book, a music stand, and a metronome. And thus began my journey.

At the same time, I was intent on writing another book, my fourth in a twenty-five year period. I reasoned that I would have more time to devote to writing now that my career as a practicing psychologist was drawing to a close. I signed up for a nonfiction writing class through the Stanford University Creative Writing Program. Desiring to sharpen my writing skills and soften my academic writing style, I was fortunate to immediately find the class I needed.

The class requirement to submit three book ideas along with the rationale for each during the first week of the class forced me to produce an outline totally off the top of my head with one option that I had never considered before. I proposed a book for those in the same life stage as myself focused on finding and expressing an art form that would, in return, benefit their brain, body, and psyche.

The juxtaposition of two disparate ideas, aging and beginning to learn, came together instantly as a book that perfectly mirrored my own experience with the Vintage Years and finding my cello.

How to Use This Book

As you begin to read *The Vintage Years,* you have some choices about how proceed. You can start at the beginning with Part I to understand how earlier life stages often get in the way of artistic expression and why it takes many of us so long to adopt an art form. Or you can begin with Part II and read the stories of more than twenty men and women who began their artistic journey after age sixty. You can begin with Part III if you want to fast-track getting started and see how the wisdom you've amassed from a lifetime of experience facilitates the learning process.

When I began researching and writing this book in earnest, I planned to interview hundreds of newbie artists and integrate their experiences in relevant chapters. What I learned from those I interviewed was so extraordinary, I couldn't bear to chop their stories into sound bites and data points. I want their stories to speak to you directly, to inspire you, and make you want to run out and explore the artist inside of you that doesn't yet have a voice or that you had to quiet in order to satisfy the demands of your earlier life.

One final note: Your artistic expression need not be limited to writing, playing a musical instrument, or the hands-on visual arts that are featured in this book. My goal was to provide a template for identifying and pursuing your creative potential and making it happen in your Vintage Years—likely the best ones for exploring and releasing your inner artist.

1   The Time of Your Life: Now or Never

Begin doing what you want to do now. We are not living in eternity.
We have only this moment, sparkling like a star in our hand-and
melting like a snowflake...
                                          —Sir Francis Bacon, 1561-1626

In 2004 a young and idealistic cello teacher living in New York City decided to do a music experiment to satisfy her curiosity. Biana Kovic thought, "I once heard that most people die with music in their heart. On hearing this statement, I felt a strong urge to do something." She quickly contacted senior residences and agencies to seek volunteers. After more than a year's search, she identified an eighty-nine-year-old woman named Matty Kahn who lived alone and independently on the upper west side of Manhattan. In the film produced to document this experiment, Matty had a youthful appearance and engaging smile. She looked eager and she energetically agreed to participate in Kovic's research.

Kovic planned to test her theory that older people could indeed learn to play music. While her students were mostly adults, she was curious about whether she could teach the cello to senior citizens, even very old ones. Kovic promised Matty Kahn a month's worth of free cello lessons in return for being the subject of this experiment. Matty was later featured in Kovic's award-winning documentary, *Virtuoso—It's Never Too Late for Cello*.

In the documentary, Matty's left hand went up and down the fingerboard playing notes, tentatively at first, and then she began naming the notes out loud as she played. She beamed with pride but seemed matter-of-fact about her playing, joking with the videographers. Her fingers betrayed her age with visible signs of arthritis, but she didn't seem deterred or in pain. A smile of satisfaction crept over her face, which deepened as she concentrated on making pleasing sounds. Not self-conscious in the least with the cameras rolling, she appeared focused on her own enjoyment as her upper body relaxed and swayed with the notes, suggesting her transcendence to a timeless and ageless place.

I wish I was privy to the thought process that led her to sign up for cello lessons. This commitment was a big departure from her day-to-day life. I wondered if it was curiosity or the desire to learn something new. Perhaps it was the recognition that time was running out and that there were some musical yearnings from her past that could still be satisfied. Maybe she wanted to take on a new challenge, or perhaps she made a bet with someone that she could do it. Likely, it was all of these and more.

Kovic's article and documentary about her elderly student learning to read music and play the cello piqued my curiosity. Although Matty's spirit of adventure may be unusual, I thought there must be other similarly curious seventy and eighty-year-olds taking on activities that nobody guessed they would embrace or could tackle. It inspired me to think about the benefits of being over fifty or sixty and taking on the study of an art form in earnest. The psychologist and scholar in me wondered if there might even be some advantages in embracing such a challenge later in life rather than in childhood or early adulthood. In fact, getting older does have benefits, and it turns out that it may be easier to learn some things *after* the age of sixty—a central theme in this book.

Matty Kahn did learn to play the cello, and it enhanced her life in several ways. It enabled her to feel masterful and proud that she could turn her life-long interest in music as a listener into performing, even if it was for an audience of one. An unanticipated outcome was the fame she experienced as the star in Kovic's documentary, which earned three film awards. In her published interview, Kovic volunteered, "I asked Matty to share some of her thoughts on two subjects that interest me the most: learning and aging. Her response was that learning keeps her going. It is the only companionship she has, especially at times when she feels lonely remembering that most of the people that she has known and loved have passed away."

While anecdotal and unscientific, Kovic and her eighty-nine-year-old student saw and experienced first hand that old brains can, in fact, do some things as well or better than twenty-year-old brains.

Sidestepping the Stereotypes

There is a popular belief, held by musicians as well as non-musicians, that the cello is a particularly difficult instrument to learn. Unlike the guitar, the cello has no frets—the ridges of wood set across a fingerboard that helps a musician's fingers to press the strings at the correct point to play a note by touch. The cello's long fingerboard on which the left hand plays notes, gives no clues as to where to place the fingers. An aspiring musician must learn to pick out the notes by feel and sound, a very subtle process. And that's just the beginning of the complexity. Beyond the difficulty of learning this instrument is the commonly held idea that musicians must start training early and the admonition, "Don't bother if you are a beginner over age ten!"

We are all familiar with the stories of child prodigies like Wolfgang Amadeus Mozart, who gave his first performance of his own compositions at age five. Like the young Mozart, artistic children who are described as geniuses reinforce the belief that great artists must start young. But the talent pool would be quite small if this adage were strictly true. The myths about musicians' ages and the value of precocity and early-identified genius were clearly irrelevant to Matty's decision.

While my curiosity about the relationship between aging and artistic interests started out as academic, I soon realized that I had a personal interest in the topic—developing my own artistic self. Up until this point in my life, if I had an inner artist, she was in a deep sleep. My interest in music was mostly limited to attending concerts and playing classical chamber music CDs. Other artistic pursuits never made it beyond the occasional museum or gallery visit.

I first learned about Kovic when I started to wonder about my own possible retirement and about the next phase of life. My forty-year career as a psychologist was devoted to helping people repair themselves and then continue developing in positive ways, but it wasn't until I began to contemplate retiring that I realized there were unexplored corners of my own life craving light and attention.

What followed was a six-month consideration of what life would look like without the work that had defined me and that had been as much a calling as a profession. Much like the clergy, psychologists have an all-encompassing sense of responsibility for their "flock." Psychologists tend not to retire early and often don't retire at all. I wrestled with the feeling that I was abandoning my patients and my profession, as if I was a quitter. Not particularly rational, part of me wanted to work until I was carried out as proof that I had given my all.

When I finally arrived at the end of my struggle, landing in resolution and relative peace, I decided to retire and began to explore the void I would be creating. Remembering Kovic's experiment fired up the aging engine inside of me. It piqued my curiosity about whether I could embark on such a journey, maybe with the added advantage of being a full twenty years younger than Matty.

I knew only too well how difficult the transition could be from working life to the life of relative leisure. Recalling some of my past clients' trepidations and fears of retirement as well as their fantasized expectations of nirvana, both extremes highly exaggerated, reminded me that I needed to do my own homework. And so I did.

The homework involved taking stock of myself at this point in life, including a review of my assets and those attributes that would get in my way. Even at a superficial level, I knew that my perseverance would serve me well and that my short attention span and self-doubt would work against me.

In anticipation of some rough going, I searched my inner and outer life for clues about any interests, long dormant or just bubbling to the surface. One that kept popping up, learning to play the cello, seemed preposterous but also intensely exciting. Being not particularly musical and post sixty-five meant the odds were very much against me, but in some way that became part of the challenge and motivation.

I would like to say that my motives were pure and that I'd always yearned to be a musician, but that would not be true. My upbringing was very practical and my family saw the fine arts as frivolous. No encouragement here.

What attracted me to the cello was its enormous size and its mellow, velvety, haunting sounds—an instrument made of beautifully polished wood that I could wrap my arms around and feel its powerful vibrations in my body when the strings were played. Quite a delicious sensation! That was a good enough reason and starting point for me.

On the other hand, I reasoned that I had finally arrived at a place in life where the daily grind would be behind me. My time would still be punctuated with routines but at a slower and less driven pace. The interests I'd cultivated in the past were still there and, while they remained satisfying, there was little to challenge me. Music, I vowed, would become my challenge and would play a bigger role in the next phase of my life.

Something had shifted inside of me. Interest in continuing to work receded and the urge to study music became stronger as my six-month exploration of retirement progressed. Deciding to make a big change in life usually means running the idea through two filters, the outside and internal world. I did just that.

The feedback from the outside world was not encouraging when I first began to talk about taking up the cello; musicians and others who claimed to have my best interests in mind thought it didn't make any sense to start at my age. Their positions mirrored their beliefs about what is possible, but I felt stereotyped and stigmatized. I believe that when they looked at me they saw an old woman, graying hair and wrinkling skin, someone like their bubbas or nanas, and without malice they reduced me to a number that suggested my irrelevancy. Maybe it was my mistake to consult younger musicians who lack the perspective that comes with age. My own adult kids were amused at my interest in taming a wild cello, not in a disrespectful way, but with surprise. They didn't seem to understand that retirement is not the last stop on the train ride.

Feedback from within myself was just as non-supportive; kind of the way adults pat little kids on the head and humor them when they say something ridiculous. I humored myself as if it was a passing fancy. I vacillated between feeling sure and unsure. I worried that I would embarrass myself, even as a student. I worried that any teacher I found would sit in judgment and think I would be more satisfied knitting a sweater than tackling a cello. I even worried about how I would lug this large wooden object around since it was more than two-thirds of my size. Seeing myself through others' eyes, especially with the critical thoughts I imbued them with, made me cringe. In my mind, a jury of nameless and faceless others disapproved of my plans and judged me harshly.

Coming of Age

In my twenties, thirties, forties, or even fifties, my perceptions of what others thought and even my own self-doubts might have made me pause, but fortunately no longer. This is a new stage in a new age. Coming of age may now refer to a number like sixty, the first point in life marked by the freedom to choose your own direction and freedom from constraints like others' needs and expectations. At this precise moment in life when a bit more time and energy is available to you, coupled with curiosity, you can invent your next life chapter. Ironically, after decades of work and the general busyness associated with managing life in the middle years, your later years may actually include more physical and creative activity than was possible when time and other resources were in short supply.

The Vintage Years is about the benefit of pursuing the life of the artist after sixty. Broadly defined, that includes writing, playing an instrument, pursuing the fine arts of one sort or another, or immersing yourself in any activity in a novel or creative way. I use the term *artist* very loosely. It's as much about the way you might approach things as the form it takes, bringing openness and a child's fascination to your experience, that which the Buddhists call "a beginner's mind."

With limited expectation of performance you can have the best possible experience for its own sake, with no worries about getting more proficient, competing with or impressing others, or having any particular goal outside of enjoyment. In fact, this is the hallmark of the over-sixty lifestyle. Not needing to prove yourself or be worried about what others think about your choices, you are finally free to explore and choose options without the nagging "shoulds" and goal-driven pressures that defined past times.

The Vintage Years is a nonfiction book. There are no made-up stories or hunches about what might be possible for you in this phase of life. The stories in subsequent chapters are about real people reinventing themselves, uncovering lost or dormant interests, or fine-tuning self-knowledge collected over a lifetime.

Many post-sixty folks volunteered to share their stories of exploration at an age that history suggests is best suited for reviewing life while sitting on the porch watching cars go by. I hope that you can identify with them so strongly that you, too, will begin to imagine yourself playing the violin or guitar. If you are not drawn to music, take a stroll through your local art supply store to see whether watercolors or pastels get you excited. Perhaps there is a secret writer in you needing inspiration or a reason to emerge. Or, your art form might be gardening, acting—anything that results in creative expression.

The Brain at Sixty

All sorts of books have been written about the years following retirement, but this book specifically focuses on the fine arts because of the benefits they provide to an aging brain, and conversely because the aging brain has capacities that actually help develop the budding, late-blooming artist. This is a circular, reinforcing process, and you are the beneficiary.

The creative arts have long been associated with the right brain: the visual/spatial and nonlinear part. The post-sixty brain is capable of using not just the right brain but also the left-brain, normally associated with a more linear, verbal, and logical function—an integration possible in the later years that makes both learning and expression more powerful. The way the brain develops and evolves with age makes it particularly suited for cre-creative expression later in life.

The burgeoning field of neuroscience, a relative newcomer to science focusing on the way the brain works, offers some good news to counterbalance the popular beliefs about the downside of getting old. Research findings suggest that humans don't outlive their quest for learning and natural curiosity. The brain, according to recent scientific research, does not simply decline, become less robust, or lose its capacity for growth. It maintains its vigor quite well and, like a muscle, if you give it exercise, it will repay your effort in some interesting ways.

Neuroscientists are in agreement that the slight increase in stress involved in learning something new actually signals the brain to make some new connections and maybe even increase neuron production. Both of these processes, which we'll come back to in some more detail later, are incredibly important to maintain optimal brain functioning and help avoid some of the deterioration that has been erroneously linked to old age.

In this age of technology, even learning to program your smart phone provides stimulation that the brain craves. Like muscles, the brain thrives on activity and use. If you practice what you enjoy, your brain will appreciate the workout and reward you in tangible ways for your efforts. If you experience passion in the process, your brain will thank you even more with sustained attention and pleasure. Just plain interest, however, is a good enough starting point to explore whatever you might want to express and to stimulate the part of you that is curious and itching to try experiencing life in a novel way.

Although the older brain shows a decrease in the density and volume of cortical gray matter, which means that it shrinks over time, it may also have the effect of producing a neural system that is more focused, specific, and efficient later in life.

These changes resulting in less gray matter can seem worrisome at first glance, but the brain is wonderfully complex and resilient, so it compensates in ways that enable the older person to actually do certain things better than was possible earlier in life. The term for this process is *neuroplasticity*, the brain's ability to adapt, renew, and reshape itself over time. This is a powerful and relatively new idea that we'll return to later. There is some evidence that over-sixty folks can actually focus better than the average young person. Our ability to zoom in on what we wish to focus on may be the compensation for other kinds of neural losses.

Neuroplasticity is not an automatic process. If you retire in the literal sense of the word, sit on the sofa or in the proverbial rocking chair watching TV, you won't be aiding your brain in its work to develop new connections, synapses, and neurons. Of course, it's unlikely you'd be reading this book if that were true for you.

Keeping neurons firing at rates that will ensure brain flexibility is an important goal that requires effort, just the kind of effort that a post-sixty is ready and able to give. Instead of being "over the hill," we might say that older people are on another hill or in the fertile valley just beyond it, looking back at the mad frenzy of life in the fast lane with some amusement.

Creativity in Abundance and Room to Grow

In his book, *The Creative Age*, psychiatrist and gerontologist Gene Cohen created the formula $C=me^2$: creativity equals a mass of knowledge multiplied by the interaction of accumulated inner and outer experience. This formula suggests that the older you get, the more your store of information and perspective on life grows, which equals creativity. Time is on your side here!

Burgeoning creativity might be the raw potential for greatness in your later years. It requires motivation and willingness to see the world and your life in new ways and to take risks that are sometimes emotionally uncomfortable, sometimes exciting, but in no way dangerous. The risks are more psychological and attitudinal, thinking outside the box of current life experience and pushing the envelope of what you think you are capable of doing. The time may be right for a new adventure, and you have the necessary tools, or at least the raw materials, to make that happen.

The tools are curiosity, openness to something new, and the willingness to try out what may seem ridiculous and absurd. You have what you need to offer to any art you choose, as well as the wisdom amassed from living on the earth and learning during all these years. What you still may need is the specific skills that come as a result of learning your heart's desire. Remember that old adage, "How do you get to Carnegie Hall? Practice, practice, practice."

Wisdom, like neuroplasticity, is another facet that may give us an edge on the young person. Elkhonon Goldberg is a neuropsychologist and author of *The Wisdom Paradox*. While his book concentrates on exploring only one aspect of the very complicated concept of wisdom, namely problem solving, he states, "Most people associate wisdom with advanced age more than anything else.... If people believe that wisdom is the privilege of old age and also regard wisdom as one of the most desirable traits then they also must believe that aging has its benefits, its positive side, and its unique and valuable assets."[1] We will see how wis-

---

[1] p. 82

dom works to override many of the purported deficits that stem from getting older.

In my research while writing this book, I came across *Lastingness: the Art of Old Age,* in which the author, Nicholas Delbanco, compares some of the world's greatest visual, literary, and musical artists in terms of those who diminish with age as opposed to those who peak as they arrive in old age. He concludes his first chapter with this statement, "Rarely—very rarely, and yet it still can happen—the final act improves upon the first."[2] It got me thinking about the final act for those of us who are not famous, or at least not yet!

It's fair to ask why I'm writing *The Vintage Years* and why now. If these many years of being a psychologist taught me anything, it is that there is a powerful life force causing us to be incredibly resilient and adaptive. This is not some mystical or spiritual argument but one based on the biological fact that all living things have strong survival instincts, and over time the best options for the species' development will be selected. Our discussion will, of course, be limited to humans and specifically to how we make the most of current physical, emotional, and cognitive resources at this point in life and how we maximize our potential. Going beyond survival basics, let's see how to thrive, manifest beauty, and leave our indelible mark on the world.

---

[2] p. 28

Being a psychologist, as well as a senior citizen, makes me aware that there are serious limitations to growth. Some of the blocks that keep a lid on possibilities for change are internal, such as self-doubt manifested in its many forms. Some are external and include the losses associated with the passage of time, or disease, or the paucity of role models in the community, or the negativity of others rooted in ageism or simply narrow-mindedness. The list goes on, and we'll explore these blocks to meeting your artistic goals and what you can do about them.

Whatever the limitations, and as long as we are alive, the potential for learning is present. Sometimes it gets lost under a pile of life's requirements and other debris. But this may be the first time in your life that you can dig out from under the mountain of to-do lists and day-to-day responsibilities to take stock and begin a new chapter.

Lifting the weight of internal and external demands and personal history can lead to feeling shell-shocked. When you're finally open to making changes in the way that you spend your time, don't run headlong into the first activity that promises to alleviate boredom or fill a void. Take the time to notice what was barely obvious before. This is the first step: to notice, observe, and take stock of the present. But getting to the present requires an understanding of the past and why it took so long to uncover our inner artist. Our search begins here.

2 Youth: The Arts Dismissed

What might be taken for a precocious genius is the genius of childhood.
—Pablo Picasso

Once, we were very young, terribly curious, bursting with energy, and open to learning—like little sponges soaking up everything in sight and without the limits eventually set by society, our families, and ourselves. Our journey to understanding the inner artist begins here. Though, for most of us, the opportunity to develop our artistry needs to wait many decades before it's finally expressed, the brain is actually quite ready in our infancy to learn any of the fine arts: drawing and painting, playing a simple instrument, or story telling in gestures, and later in writing.

When you were born, although you won't remember this, someone very likely held you, rocked you, and sang to you. Whether it was a lullaby, gentle humming, or melodic whispering, it probably helped you to feel relaxed, safe, and nurtured. There was little else demanding attention in that time of life, and your five senses soaked up every experience. You quickly absorbed what you heard, saw, touched, tasted, and smelled. Your grownups understood this intuitively, so they hung colorful, gyrating, and maybe musical mobiles over your crib to stimulate and entertain you. They understood that these measures would be good for you in some way—either to calm and soothe you or maybe even to increase your intelligence.

Memories before the age of three are so rare that it won't be easy to recall yourself back then, but picture any baby or toddler, and you can see the young brain at work. Toddlers are always busy using their senses to explore the world. What is lost to us or glossed over for expediency is novel and even exciting to a young child. The smallest sound doesn't escape their attention. The smallest object or speck of dirt beckons notice and even manipulation. There is no end to their fascination with everything that can be experienced through their sense of smell, touch, sound, vision, and taste.

I'm thinking about my twin grandsons who were twenty months old when I shared the following experience with them. After their naps, when the twins were alert and brimming with energy, I packed up the car and drove them to the local YWCA for their weekly, one-hour class designed for the under-two-year-old learner.

The room was outfitted with all sorts of tempting playthings arranged in a seemingly random way. Little brightly colored cars and balls sat waiting for eager hands. Stuff to crawl over, climb on, and jump upon encircled the perimeter of the room. Pint-size percussion instruments like drums, cymbals, bells, tambourines, and cucarachas were strewn about on the floor. A sticky tack cloth covered one wall, while felt shapes in various colors sat in a pile on the floor beneath it, waiting for an artistic placement.

While I found the room to be a little chaotic and over-stimulating for my aging brain, it was just right for a not-quite-two-year-old.

The psychologist in me was curious about how the dozen or so waddlers (so called because they are not quite toddlers) would choose activities. It didn't take long to find out. The musical instruments were a hit. While little fingers pounded and shook them, in the center of the floor little feet danced around to the music. Some waddlers watched, sitting and swaying to the sounds. A few drifted over to the sticky board and began to pick felt pieces from the stack on the floor. These eager artists made decisions about sizes, shapes, colors, and placement, creating bright and interesting pictures. Of course, a limited attention span made this a short-lived activity.

Later, an organized activity led by the teacher consisted of a group song with accompanying hand and body movements. The parents and waddlers seemed familiar with the arrangements, and I tried to lip-synch to both fit in and try to fathom what they might be feeling. I imagine that weekly repetition of the same songs, such as the old standby, "When you're happy and you know it clap your hands," gives the kids a sense of mastery and forms a sort of oral story that they can repeat and understand. Their smiles and focused attention suggested true pleasure and possibly some real understanding of this activity. Indeed, in the following days and weeks, the same songs and gestures were repeated many times by the twins at home with an attempt to get participation by their parents and grandma. It was a form of communication that was understood all around and that the twins could initiate.

As the class ended, the parents gathered up their kids and all of the requisite paraphernalia, heading out in different directions until the next week. This is just a snippet of a young child's life in California in the twenty-first century.

I am cautious about extrapolating this experience to all young children or even to all preschoolers in the United States. But it is true that very little ones everywhere delight in hitting a pot with two sticks to make music, or drawing with a twig in the sand or dirt outside their dwelling. It has been this way from the beginning of time.

Baby Brain

It is no accident that the human brain is primed for music, visual art, and symbols that later develop into writing. In the first few years after birth, the brain goes through a period of very rapid neural development. These neurons are like building blocks that form the basis of our memories. More than at any other time in our lives, the infant brain is actively making neural connections and building structures that are foundational to further learning. By the time we reach the age of eight or ten, the brain is already pruning these connections to keep only the most important and frequently used ones. The brain detests clutter! The art, music, and writing experienced to that point create a foundation for our further understanding and interest. It remains for a lifetime, patiently waiting to be tapped. Very often youth doesn't offer an opportunity for the artist to flourish.

Daniel Levitin, neuroscientist, musician, and author of *This Is Your Brain On Music*, emphasizes the importance of music to the very young, absorptive, and pliable brain. "Basic structural elements are incorporated into the very wiring of our brains when we listen to music early in our lives. . . . Our brain imposes structure and order on a sequence of sounds. Just how this structure leads us to experience emotional reactions is part of the mystery of music"[3]. The connection between music and emotion is very strong and learned early in life. You might be able to remember music from your early childhood, and it's likely associated with positive emotions. These memories can even predate memories associated with spoken language.

A case in point: When my daughter was a baby, the movie *Chariots of Fire* aired in a neighborhood theater. Taking advantage of her naptime and to avoid the cost of a babysitter, we took her with us. She slept through most of the show but seemed alert and awake from time to time. The sound track from this movie was very compelling and emotionally moving, at least in my opinion.

Many years later, when we heard the sound track played on the radio, the same daughter, then probably a teen, stopped to listen very intently—in a way that teens reserve for very few things. She said she knew that piece of music and had heard it many times in her head but didn't know why. Following the trail, we wound up back in her late infancy, long before she could talk or consciously remember much. She had warm and very positive associations with the music, which was clearly coupled with sleeping in a cozy place on her mom's lap. In fact, the music by Greek composer Vangelis became more famous than the Academy Award-winning film itself.

Daniel Levitin describes his own early experience: "One of my earliest memories of music is as a three-year-old, lying on the floor underneath the family's grand piano as my mother played. Lying on our shaggy green wool carpet, with the piano above

---

[3] p. 107

me, all I could see were my mother's legs moving the pedals up and down, but the sound—it engulfed me! It was all around, vibrating through the floor and through my body, the low notes to the right of me, the high notes to the left. The loud, dense chords of Beethoven; the flurry of dancing, acrobatic notes of Chopin; the strict, almost militaristic rhythms of Schumann, a German like my mother. In these—among my first memories of music—the sound held me in a trance; it transported me to sensory places I had never been. Time seemed to stand still while the music was playing".[4]

Music seems to have the capacity to tap into the primitive brain structure where emotions, and especially the experience of pleasure, reside. Because music is such a source of delight for even very young children, listening, playing music, and using instruments to make pleasant sounds is highly reinforcing. It is analogous to giving a young child, or any of us for that matter, something delicious to eat. We crave more of what tastes good because the positive sensation and any subsequent tasting of the treat evokes a similar, very positive emotion. In other words, we get hooked.

Listening to music and playing musical instruments activate several regions of the brain and result in a number of cognitive and emotional outcomes, especially the experience of pleasure. This is caused by the release of endorphins, which are the body's natural pain relievers and mood enhancers. Structurally similar to opioids, when released in the brain, endorphins lead to feelings of well-being. If the word *opioid* sounds familiar, it may be because it identifies a category of substances, including opium,

---

[4] p. 129

which are responsible for certain drug addictions.

The take-away idea here is not about drug addiction but about the pleasures that the arts provide, stimulating the same regions of the brain as endorphins. In general, we tend to seek out what gives us pleasure—and the arts have the capacity to do this. It's no surprise that music improves people's moods and can even produce euphoria.

Viewing and expressing visual art seems to have the same emotional effect as playing music. Activity deep within the primitive part of the brain, sometimes referred to as the reptilian brain, causes this feel-good experience. The so-called reptilian brain preceded the more sophisticated parts of the brain, relatively recent additions within the past fifty thousand years. Our very remote ancestors took pleasure from music and art, which evoked strong emotions.

Visual art, unlike music, activates a different part of the brain called the visual cortex. Although story telling through written language occurs at a developmentally later stage, my twenty-month old grandsons can tell a richly detailed story through hand signals and gestures sprinkled with just a few words. When their tales are understood and appreciated they are very likely to do more. Perhaps there are born storytellers in us all.

If it is in our nature and we're born to create stories, music, and art, why is that so, and why is it so important? To answer those questions we need to explore our collective history as a species, which takes us back into our primordial past.

In The Very Beginning of Time

We can speculate about the importance of the arts to our early ancestors back when survival meant outrunning or outsmarting a mastodon at the cave entrance, but some hard evidence of its significance actually exists.

Darwin's theory of evolution helps explain why species developed along certain lines. Those strategies that proved to be effective in survival were passed along to subsequent generations in terms of genetic changes. This theory is not limited to physical characteristics but extends to brain function as well. In evolutionary terms, what was useful to survival became hardwired in the brain and the rest became obsolete. On an individual level, remember that the brain avoids clutter, and just like pruning the apple tree, brain pruning makes what's left more robust.

Evolutionary psychology, a relatively new field of study, and its cadre of scientists who study the brain, investigate how and why cognitive functioning evolved from the beginning of humanoid time. It turns out that how we see and experience the world are products of an evolutionary process spanning more than one hundred thousand years.

But what exactly is the survival value of music, art, and telling stories through writing? In answering that question, we need to start with a huge generalization and an over-simplification.

It is likely that one of the qualities differentiating humans from other living organisms is our ability to understand mortality, which can be very burdensome without explanations that are calming and reassuring. This is the role typically played by spirituality in general and religion more specifically. One hypothesis suggests that in the very beginning of time, the rituals created by music, art, and storytelling satisfied our need to know about the hereafter by providing some emotional soothing and hope that made everyday life more predictable, explainable, and even tolerable.

The elders in the tribe, worn down by the passage of time and the harshness of daily life, were no longer very useful in hunting or gathering. But they had the knowledge of the species stored in their heads, passed down through stories, rituals, visual images, dances, and sounds made on bone instruments and animal-skin drums. They were the wise ones who had the maturity and judgment as well as the storehouse of knowledge. We will return to the role of the wise elders later in the book when we explore the Vintage Years and Wisdom to see how art, music, and writing use the benefits of hardwiring to flourish and impact the later years.

"Some of the oldest human-made artifacts found at archaeological sites are musical instruments. Music is important in the daily lives of most people in the world, and has been throughout human history," states Levitin in *The World in Six Songs*.[5] He suggests music's universality across time and space and goes on to say, "Our urge toward artistic expression shows up in cave paintings and decorations . . . such as thirty-thousand year-old water jugs. Some of the earliest cave paintings show humans dancing".[6]

Levitin also makes a case for the primacy of music, predating spoken language, and maybe contributing to the formation of language. It makes me think about the waddlers I recently spent time with, none of whom spoke except for some isolated

---

[5] p. 2
[6] p. 20

nouns accompanied by much gesturing. All of them had the capacity to experience and express rhythm and movement through song, dance, and playing instruments, albeit toy ones. "There is no tangible evidence that language preceded music," says Levitin. "In fact, the physical evidence suggests the contrary. Music is no doubt older than the fifty-thousand-year-old bone flute, because flutes were unlikely the first instruments".[7]

In the beginning of human time, the arts bound together the past and the future, the everyday and the unknown world of the spirit, and the youngest and oldest members of the clan. That was the arts' survival value, and as the evolutionary psychologists might say, that is why the arts and our attunement to them were selected as traits to become hardwired genetically. The arts made sense out of our existence as well as offering an emotional outlet for our joys, pain, suffering, and unanswerable questions.

That was all long ago—theories based on artifacts and assumptions. But look at any baby or young child available to you. Play music and watch baby's movement. Show a visual and watch baby's fascination with it. Tell a story with gestures and notice baby's tracking of it. Look back into your own distant past. Remember your own experiences: your first memory of song or music; your first music making with whatever materials were at hand; your first story acted out with props and dance-like movement. What do you recall of it? What emotions does it evoke? The young child-artist in you is still alive and well, a free spirit unencumbered by rules and roles, waiting to be liberated. But not liberated in your youth.

---

[7] p. 250

The School Years

If the arts are so good for the brain and are hardwired because of their usefulness to survival, why do they get all but extinguished during childhood, adolescence, and young adulthood?

The years of formal education give structure to eager, energetic, and curious youngsters. School can also stifle the creative spirit. It's not designed to do that but certainly can and often does produce those results. It is a time of socialization and learning the rules for navigating a world filled with others' needs and demands. Creative thought and expression require thinking outside of the box, which necessitates not fitting into the boxes that school and society at large require in order to avoid standing out as an oddity.

David Kelley, the preeminent American product designer who established the global design consultancy IDEO, the d.school (Hasso Plattner Institute of Design) at Stanford University, and is credited with introducing the concept of design thinking, believes that all kids have the natural capacity for creativity, that is, "at least until the educational system beats it out of them".[8] He works with students at Stanford to retrain the right side of the brain; often dormant for a decade or two during which time the goal-oriented left-brain is fed by society's or parents' demands. The college-age students he works with have lost only a few years to the linear thinking that is prevalent during the school years—learn this, memorize that.

For example, meet Betsy whose story appears in Part II of this book. Some of her fondest memories were of summer camp

---

[8] *Fast Company Magazine*; February 1, 2009

where she played with clay and paper, fashioning them into three-dimensional objects to enjoy and wear. At school, that kind of activity was not only considered frivolous but an interference with the serious work of a girl who would later become a scientist. At the time, she didn't think much about it. The fun and pleasure associated with her artistic curiosity had nothing to do with the important stuff: performing well enough to please her parents and others who would guide her career path. Only now, as an artist in her sixties, does she look back with nostalgia mixed with chagrin for the lost play.

When Gene was a young child, he looked forward to spending time in his cousin's basement where he watched and admired the young adult standing at an easel. Fascinated by the oils and particularly the smell of the paints, he still has olfactory memories tied to these experiences. He wished painting could fit into his schedule, but his perceived lack of talent and a busy inner-city lifestyle, coupled with his father's practicality, got in the way. It took fifty years to actually put himself in his cousin's shoes.

As a child of the Depression and poverty, Yvette spun tales that became plays for the neighborhood kids. She wrote limericks and kept a diary as a girl, and showed promise as a writer, which was recognized by her high school guidance counselor. But the need for money and the war years conspired to end her education when she was only fifteen. That was the end of putting on paper the musings of her imagination until a chance long-distance railroad trip in her late fifties breathed new life into her writing.

The school years offer creative opportunities for some children who show talent, or have artistic role models, or have mentors who nurture the young artist's interest. The rest of us generally had exposure to art and music in kindergarten. If we were lucky and attended a well-endowed school, we may have had access to dedicated classes or perhaps an orchestra. But that may not be enough to foster a lifelong interest in and practice of an art form because of the mounting pressure from competing activities like sports, academic requirements, a part-time job, or just hanging out.

Those who studied a musical instrument in their childhood often report it was under duress by parents who meant well but took a hard-nosed approach to practicing and other rules. One young student took up the oboe, because that instrument was available in music class, when he really wanted to play a trumpet. It soured him toward playing an instrument for a long time.

Reflecting on their past experiences with the arts as children, some of the people I interviewed were mocked by their friends or siblings and labeled uncool because they preferred to paint or write stories while their less arty friends spent time washing their cars or talking on the phone. There may be examples from your life as well.

Darya, whom we will also meet in Part II, had an extraordinarily strong emotional reaction to color, even as a three-year-old. Life steered her away from art until age fifty-eight, and during our interview she looked back with some longing at the missed opportunity to study art formally when she was young. The road not taken can never be known, but the one she took did meet her needs at the time. She shrugged when we spoke about it, as if she was trying to shake off the idea and put it into a perspective that gave her some comfort. "Oh well, if I'd done that, I would have probably burned out early anyway."

Of course, colleges have music, art, and creative-writing departments. Some students have enough interest, talent, and perseverance, and do in fact make careers out of the arts. They try to beat the odds of becoming a starving artist, a label that is daunting and at the same time undermining. The history of the arts is replete with names of artists who did succeed—and we're grateful for their tenacity and genius. We'll meet some of these famous late bloomers in Part III. But, this book is about those of us whose art didn't blossom until much later in life.

3 Adulthood: The Arts Postponed

Adults are obsolete children.

—Dr. Seuss

On an overcast Sunday afternoon in Hanolai Bay, Hawaii, a small crowd gathered in the local community center for a slack key guitar concert. This kind of music is indigenous to the Hawaiian Islands and helps explain how childlike naiveté and curiosity can lead to creating a new musical form.

Sandy and Doug McMaster aren't the typical music duet. They are husband and wife of more than thirty years, musicians, musicologists, and legends in Hawaii. The first time I saw them was ten years ago on the beach where they held court about once a week and played music as the sun set. Locals and tourists drifting by were captured by the music, free to all who chose to sit on the beach facing the ocean and the setting sun. To the uninitiated and those trained in traditional European style music, the sound was a bit jolting, but the curious stayed to have the experience, which like the Islands, was calming and peaceful.

Where did this music come from and why is it important to a book about finding your inner artist later in life? The way the slack key guitar evolved provides a rich example of what is possible when adults maintain their childlike curiosity and openness to learning, facilitated by a simple life. This is not really possible in twenty-first-century developed countries where adulthood is mostly confined to adult pursuits. What follows is the story about how this music came to be.

Interspersed among the lilting, melodic songs passed down through generations of families and interpreted by Doug McMaster, Sandy McMaster explained the history of this art form in her almost trance-like style. Sandy is one of those people whose voice and gestures evoke a calmness and well-being so compelling that before you know it, as an audience member, you find yourself relaxing and breathing more slowly. She served as the narrator for the twosome, chronicling the local history of slack key guitar music.

In the 1780s, Hawaii's King Kamehameha received an unusual gift, presumably from Captain James Cook who landed his two ships off the coast of Kauai. The present, a herd of cattle—previously unknown to the natives—roamed the Hawaiian plains and grew in size. Lush from frequent rain and full of nutrients, the land turned out to be compatible with bovine well-being, and the cattle multiplied to the point of overrunning the taro and rice crops, which were the mainstay diet of the Hawaiian people. While this is an example of how too much of a good thing is not so good, the locals valued the abundance but realized a need for a better way to manage the cattle's free-range lifestyle.

Mexican cowboys signed on to an adventure and sailed to Kauai from what is probably now California, maybe coming from as far as Arizona, Colorado, or New Mexico. Since their contracts required a couple of years' commitment and leaving their families behind, they brought their guitars to keep them company and ease their longings. This simple gesture, through a number of accidental and serendipitous events, led to the creation of a new musical genre known as slack key guitar.

The indigenous people of Hawaii had music, but since they were so isolated from other civilizations, it was homegrown and not influenced by formal music theory. Instruments were made from whatever grew on the land: gourds and trees. So, you might say that it was rich in percussion music: drums and rattles of all kinds plus flutes made from reeds. Stringed instruments, like the guitar, had not been seen before this time and were curiosities indeed. The cowboys did not intend to entertain the locals, but played in the evenings to soothe themselves, to stay connected to their homelands, and to sing about the families and lives they left behind.

But the locals were mesmerized and drawn to the music and the instruments, which had their origin in seventeenth-century Spain. Because music is so much a language hardwired into the human species from the beginning of time, its universality was the common denominator that drew the cowboys and Hawaiians together. First were the spontaneous jam sessions: Mexican guitars and Hawaiian percussions. Then came the teaching and learning and cross-pollinating that resulted over time. And so it was that the natives learned to play the guitar.

What follows is the account of how playing the guitar led to what is known as the slack key guitar. It came about as a problem-solving act born in frustration. When the cowboys left, they gave their guitars as gifts to the local families whom they had come to know and love. What they didn't leave was a method for tuning the guitars, which the cowboys knew intuitively but didn't pass along as a set of instructions. It didn't take long for the instruments to require tuning as rain and humidity caused the wood to swell and affect the sound of the strings.

The Spanish guitar tuning method was lost, and the Hawaiians' adjustments to the strings produced new sounds, equally pleasant to local taste, but not conventional to a trained Western music ear. The new sound wasn't standardized. Different families found their own tuning and created their own music and words, usually about life on the Islands and things they saw: flowers, sunsets, features of the land, and emotions like love.

Beautiful music, with no standard or set of immutable rules, guided by instinct and internal senses, led to a profusion of sounds that were reminiscent of the Mexicans but suited to the island pace. Slack key guitar playing was born. Later, the ukulele was created, tuned like the slack key guitar, and often accompanied it as the trademark Hawaiian style.

Creativity Inhibited

The Hawaiian sound developed out of curiosity, problem solving, and the absence of clear-cut, well-articulated rules that might have interfered with its creation. First came the fascination with the Mexican cowboys playing their foreign-sounding instruments. Then came the problem of tuning it after the cowboys left their guitars behind. Next came the process of trial and error, experimenting without a goal in mind. Then came the feeling of pleasure and satisfaction, created by making a pleasant sound and remembering the feeling and the way it came about. Nobody said, "No, that isn't the way to play music," or, "That sounds terrible," or, "You should or shouldn't do it this way."

No music rules and no authorities to follow: this is the formula for stimulating creativity.

Now let's explore the aspects of life that inhibit creativity and help explain why, for many of us, playing an instrument, writing a story, or painting a picture often does not happen until we are sixty.

Going way back to the age of majority, currently eighteen, and until near-retirement or late fifties, we are discouraged in many ways from pursuing the arts. Of course, some of us do embrace the arts at a young age despite the warnings inherent in the phrase *starving artist*, and some of us even become household names like Picasso and Mozart. Since you are reading this book, you are not likely an early-identified artist.

Eighteen years of age marks the beginning of adulthood in the United States, when you accept most of the privileges and responsibilities that come with this status. It's assumed that your judgment is sufficiently mature to make informed decisions, so you are able to vote, marry, join the armed forces, and buy cigarettes. You may be able to drive a car at sixteen or younger, depending on the state.

While physical development is mostly complete by eighteen, men and some women continue to grow taller until their mid-twenties, and wisdom teeth seldom surface before this time. Brain development is another story. The prefrontal cortex, evolutionarily the most recently developed part of the brain, is still a work in progress. Still, by age eighteen, most young people are headed for college or the work force, and at least theoretically, are ready for adult life and its challenges.

Society has a modicum of hope that its youth can manage most things when they are turned loose on the world at eighteen. The irony is that most newly minted adults are pretty sure that their judgment is sufficient whereas, at age fifty they would likely be amazed, in retrospect that they survived at all. Nevertheless, most of us do survive our youthful choices and indiscretions.

We are sufficiently socialized to not stand out enough to garner push back by our peers or authorities like the police or dean of students. Our bad behavior tends to be within limits, which is the good news. Our behavior in general, as well as attitudes about most things, is also confined to the acceptable rules of living. While this prevents anarchy, it can also strangle or at least curtail uniqueness and creativity, which is the bad news.

Living life within the parameters of cultural expectations is easier than pushing the envelope. We all want to stand out somewhat, but not too much, which can lead to negative attention from peers, family, or some authority. Life at this stage has all kinds of challenges and paradoxes: make your mark on the world, but do it within legal limits; compete to be your best, but don't flaunt it, and be sensitive to others' feelings; be your own personal best, but fit in by having a lifestyle that's acceptable to our culture at any point in time.

Until eighteen, and even more likely until our early or mid twenties, we take in information about the world and ourselves, rehearsing what we learn within safe limits. Then, adulthood provides the opportunity to practice what we've learned until that point—this is prime time, the live performance with consequences!

Unique, But Not Quite

Individually, we create a life that is seemingly unique and fits our physical, psychological, and intellectual boundaries. We may set goals or flounder our way into work and social situations, making mistakes along the way for sure, but believing that even these mistakes are unique to us. And so they are—to some extent.

In truth, we are not as free as we imagine and would like to believe. I'm not talking about the old argument of free will verses determinism. Regardless of your religious beliefs about this, adulthood is a fairly structured stage of life determined only in part by your unique personhood. The brain determines the developmental tasks that are hardwired into the human species and much of what happens in adulthood. In other words, the successful completion of adulthood depends on accomplishing the goals of adulthood. While they aren't handed to us in a bound notebook, they are somehow learned and mostly satisfied.

The multiple jobs of adulthood seem to inhibit the very kind of explorations that led to the creation of slack key guitar in Kauai, in a faraway time and place where rules for adult living were not so narrowly defined.

The Life Stage Called Adulthood

Unless you were a psychology major in college, you may not know much about how adulthood was defined by psychologists like Erik Erikson, who was a pioneer in the field of developmental psychology. His groundbreaking theory of developmental stages in the first half of the twentieth century was accurate as far as it went, but sadly left the years north of forty mostly un-chartered.

The collective sentiment of scholars and scientists, even in the 1950s, was that bothering with the years past forty was a waste of time, as growth ceased and decline began at that point. This view is partly true, of course, in that physical decline does begin before the age of thirty, and the brain's processing speed also begins to decline at about that time. Still, it is false for the most part, because we now know that psychological growth and brain development do continue well into old age, as we shall see as we read on.

Erikson's stages are important nevertheless, not for prescriptive purposes because few of us want to live our lives by the book, but for understanding the scope of a twenty-year cycle that we all pass through in one way or another to arrive at the Vintage Years.

No matter how you lived your adult years, when you accomplish certain goals you prevent others from happening. No one has enough bandwidth to do it all. That is what this book is about: finding your passion, your inner artist, when the demands of adulthood are finally satisfied.

How Adulthood Constrains the Inner Artist

The years from twenty to forty encompass an extraordinarily busy time, as I'm sure you recall. During the first twenty years, the focus of life is on acquisition of knowledge about the world, development of the body and development of the brain, including its capacity to grow, organize, and sort through a sea of data. Much of this happens without our conscious attention. What we learn is guided by what we attend to and the local landscape of our individual lives. But how we learn is determined by factors generally not under our control including idiosyncratic learning styles and disabilities.

By twenty, we look sufficiently like adults and have the necessary building blocks in place to take on the challenges of adult life, more or less. As I write these words, the psychologist in me wants to say, "Yes, but so much goes on during the first twenty formative years that I really can't gloss over and summarize so quickly." I remind myself that this isn't a book on developmental psychology, and that you aren't reading it to get a comprehensive picture of how your brain and body mastered childhood, adolescence, and early adulthood. But I do want to provide you with a rationale for the delayed expression of your inner artist, which may have had to wait until sixty to finally get your time and attention.

While the timelines have changed over the past hundred years, the developmental tasks of the decades between twenty and forty or fifty have to do with becoming established in a job, developing interpersonal relationships leading to a special bond, and perhaps getting married or pairing with another person and raising a family.

A hundred years ago, most of these milestones would likely have been accomplished by the late teens or early twenties, but these days the mid or late forties might be a more reasonable estimate. The trajectory to full adulthood is much longer these days, partly due to an extended period of education, the broadened role of women which extends the childbearing years, and the economy which may make it more difficult for young adults to become financially independent.

At the evolutionary level, all of us humans have approximately the same job: to survive to adulthood, procreate, protect our young so that they can survive to adulthood, find a way to keep our bodies alive by feeding it, and keeping it safe, and join with others in a social community for mutual benefit. There it is, our life boiled down to its most basic form and having little to do with us as individuals.

Our individual lives follow this template for the most part, but there are innumerable possible combinations of factors that create our uniqueness and specialness. Just a few of the determining factors include: where and how we grew up—farm or city; rich or poor; male or female; our family constellation; our culture; luck or other life circumstances, educational level achieved, personality, health and a long, long list of others.

Erik Erikson, the developmental psychologist referenced earlier, led a long life that spanned almost all of the twentieth century. He suggested that our course of development is determined by an interaction of the body (genetic biological programming), the mind (psychological), and cultural influences. Of course, I am summarizing volumes of psychological, philosophical, and neurological ideas in this oversimplified taxonomy in order to convey how adulthood inhibited the devel-development of the inner artist.

Erikson's psychosocial theory of development has eight stages encompassing the years from birth to death. A summary follows with the conflicts that he says need to be resolved and which are characteristic of the various adult stages:

- Young adulthood spans the years between nineteen and forty. The key conflict is Intimacy vs. Isolation, and the challenge is developing intimacy with someone to avoid isolation.

• Middle adulthood generally occurs between ages forty and sixty-five. During this stage, work is most crucial, as well as the issues that surround family life. If we are ever to experience being in charge or being in control, this is the stage when this long–wished-for role might take place. Generativity vs. Stagnation is pinpointed as the relevant conflict that needs to be satisfied by giving forward to the next generation. Like other stages we've described, generativity happens closer to sixty-five, since these days some folks are just getting started in their adult lives at forty. We'll focus on generativity in the chapter on Wisdom.

• Maturity, as a stage, takes place after sixty-five. Erikson describes the conflict as Ego Integrity vs. Despair. According to Erikson, it is a time of reflection on one's life and whether it was well lived. If the conclusion comes up negative, then despair is the outcome. A *fait accompli*, at this point, it seems that there is little for a person to do in order to grow or make changes. This is Erikson's idea, a reflection of the limited perspective of pre-twenty-first-century thinking!

Necessary Distractions

During my research for this book, and based on conversations with numerous individuals who were still ten years away from Medicare benefits, as well as those thirty years into retirement, I saw a pattern that wasn't surprising but nevertheless striking in its consistency. I always asked the people I interviewed why their artistry waited in the wings of their lives until age fifty-five, or sixty-eight, or seventy-nine. Unfailingly, I heard, "I was busy making a living," or, "Between work, wife, kids, and taking care of a home, I barely had time to think about anything else," or, "I traveled too much for work; I had no down time." These answers focused on very limited time and competing demands from society and family.

The early adult years are about finding a job or career and climbing the relevant ladders, because getting ahead is one of the achievement goals of the age period between twenty and forty-five. Whether the goal was personal or an expectation of family or society is not so relevant now that it is in the past. Still, most of us hopped on this merry-go-round because we felt good when we succeeded and, frankly, there were few positive alternatives. Psychologically speaking, as Erikson's developmental stages detailed, early and mid adulthood are spent in the search for intimacy with another person or within a community and on making a mark on the world.

Although Erik Erikson provided a theory that worked for the twentieth century, it didn't go far enough to explain the goals and challenges of middle and late adulthood. Gene Cohen, a psychiatrist and gerontologist who authored two seminal books in the first decade of the twenty-first century, spent his whole career studying and interviewing thousands of older adults. He had quite a bit to say about the later stages of psychosocial development.

The first of Cohen's stages usually occurs between the early forties and late fifties. He refers to this stage as "midlife reevaluation" wherein the sense of mortality surfaces and influences our lives for the first time. When the awareness of one's own mortality appears, it ushers in a new depth of human experience. In fact, philosophers and scientists suggest that humans may be the only species that can imagine their own death, affecting their decisions and choices in significant ways for the rest of their lives. Out of this awareness comes a growing interest in making the remaining years count in ways not possible before.

The preciousness of time in adulthood may prevent us from exploring ways to enhance meaning. Making changes consistent with the pull of mortality needs to wait for a later stage. Cohen points out that "brain changes during this phase spur developmental intelligence, which is the basis for wisdom," which emerges in a later phase of development.[9]

Biologically-Driven Inhibitors

Erikson and Cohen focused on the psychosocial development during adulthood, but physiologically, there is a different picture. As the brain matures in early adolescence, when secondary sex characteristics become apparent, girls and boys take on the appearance of men and women and produce hormones that greatly affect behavior, perception of the world, and self-expression.

The brain signals the manufacture of estrogen and testosterone in proportion to gender, with males producing more testosterone and females more estrogen. But females do produce some testosterone, and some estrogen can be found in men. Overlap may actually help reduce misunderstandings between the sexes, since at the purely physical level, very masculine men and hyper feminine women would have almost nothing in

---

[9] *The Mature Mind*; p. 52

common. Mother nature may not have had that in mind, but it does help in cross-gender communication, which is complicated enough!

Estrogen and testosterone exert a powerful drive at the physical level—surging and propelling adolescent development, maintaining a steady state through adulthood, and then decreasing sometime between the age of fifty and sixty.

What, you might be wondering, does this have to do with the inhibition of the inner artist during adulthood? Quite a bit, actually. Anders Greenwood, Ph.D., is a neuropsychologist and colleague with whom I consulted about this very subject. As we ate our lunches in a busy Palo Alto restaurant, I picked his brain about the ways an older brain facilitates the creation and expression of the inner artist. He suggested that as testosterone production decreases in men as they age, a more relaxed and calmer person emerges.

The drives that characterize early and middle male adulthood—achievement, intense competition, procreation, and protecting the family—give way to more openness in experiencing and expressing meaning and emotion. At this stage, there is a shift of attention to non-biologically-driven goals, those that are truly unique and are not accomplished to satisfy life's demands.

The process is similar for women in that estrogen, like in other species, causes women to focus attention first and foremost on bonding with a partner, building a nest, creating a family, and insuring its survival. Remember, we are talking here only about the physiological pull, which leaves out the drives toward other more complex processes that human brains are capable of and do in abundance during adulthood.

Both Dr. Greenwood and I realize that while the purely physiological explanation is a gigantic oversimplification, when you examine the hormone-driven behaviors that men and women share with other animals, and mammals in particular, you get a species very focused on accomplishing the mandates of adulthood with little room for much else.

Never Too Late

There you have it. Adulthood really isn't the time in life for most of us to adopt art. There's just not the bandwidth, the neurological or the cognitive focus. The good news is that The Vintage Years more than balance the scale. With your decades of life experience mounting and your perceptions rich and deep by the end of this stage, you now enter a long phase, ripe and ready from the seeds planted long ago, in your earliest days.

The pace has slowed. Hormones are steadier. Keeping up with any standards that seemed exceedingly important before is a thing of the past. It's time now to see the broader picture, to take in what was not possible previously. The artist's prime time is here.

4   The Vintage Years: The Arts Embraced

I have reached an age when, if someone tells me to wear socks, I don't have to.

—Albert Einstein

The Vintage Years encompass the vast, open time frame beyond the noisy and hectic periods that preceded them. As the metaphor in Chapter 1 suggested, rather than going over the hill into oblivion or decrepitude, the Vintage Years are like the fertile valley on the other side with potential that isn't really noticeable until you see it up close. No doubt there will be challenges, particularly physical—and sometimes cognitive—slowing, but the trade-off, according to research, is greater satisfaction and generally improved mood. This valley is where your inner artist receives the nourishment to come to life.

I want to shout to the world, having crossed the threshold into this stage myself, that it is loaded with opportunity for growth and self-appreciation, and for expression that hasn't been possible before. This is truly act three in life, where it all comes together, like a stage play in which the final act resolves conflicts and finishes on a high note. But it wasn't always this way.

When the twentieth century began, the average lifespan for men was forty-six and for women, forty-eight. By the beginning of the twenty-first century, only one hundred years later, the average lifespan was seventy-four for men and eighty for women. Quite a jump, you might say, but simply adding years to a life is not the best measure of a life well lived. Adding quantity but not quality brings to mind a rather dismal image of oldsters sitting in dingy nursing homes staring at nothing in particular or watching endless hours of TV.

This scenario often did unfold without much challenge until nearly the end of the twentieth century, partly because of limited good role models of successful aging, and partly due to almost no research detailing what works well in the last third of life. It didn't help that the life span was shorter and the concept of a three-decade retirement didn't exist. These limiting ideas were replaced only recently, and there's no need to dwell on the stereotypes as we are only too cognizant of them and their affect on policies and perceptions of seniors.

Life Beyond Myths and Roles

By the end of the first decade of the twenty-first century, the baby boomers, known for their take-charge and activist approach to life, began to reach retirement age and collectively were not content to sit on their porches and rock in their rocking chairs. The media began to take notice and depicted retirees as energetic and interested in a fuller and more exciting life. Ads in print media, on TV, and now on wireless gadgets show gray-haired but youthful seniors doing what pleases them, free from earlier restrictions and with more available time.

The American Association of Retired Persons, better known as *AARP*, publishes a couple of magazines and has a strong lobby to champion the rights of seniors. Scanning recent issues of the *AARP Bulletin* reveals the focus is mostly on health, disease management, financial planning, retirement planning in general, and solving the problems of aging. It portrays today's elders as involved and brimming with interest. Some attention, though not nearly enough, goes to the budding creativity that can be the hallmark of the Vintage Years. Our society still has a way to go in depicting seniors as the wise elders we are, enhanced by a lifetime of walking the earth, enabled by our capacity for further development. That is the legacy of the Vintage Years.

No one would deny that getting older brings limitations, but aging per se doesn't lead to disease nor are most diseases associated with aging. Even when there are constraints caused by a disease process, whether physical or cognitive, the richness of accumulated life experience, leading to what we commonly refer to as wisdom, continues to offset the losses. We'll focus on wisdom explicitly in Chapter 8.

Remember the plasticity of the brain—modifiable and adaptable. "There's plasticity from cradle to grave.... The brain learns what it's got to do at the time,"[10] states Norman Doidge, M.D., psychiatrist and author of *The Brain That Changes Itself*. "This is the most fantastic part: what you think and imagine can actually change the structure of the brain, down to the very connections between the brain cells.... Learning changes the number of con-

---

[10] Interview with Allan Gregg on *Science Friday*; TV Ontario, 10/25/10

nections between the neurons, the nerve cells in the nervous system."[11]

New Interest in the Aging Brain

Thanks to the technological developments in the last quarter of the twentieth century, the computer became a workhorse in all kinds of settings that benefit aging baby boomers. At about this same time, coincidentally but not accidentally, the scientific community began to make breakthroughs in further understanding how the brain functions as well as its potential to modify itself in several positive ways. Studies of the brain, previously impossible before now, garnered attention. Enter the new discipline of the cognitive neuroscience of aging that depended on very new methods for measuring the brain's activity.

Just to give you an idea of the extensiveness of these measures, here is a list of imaging techniques used to study a person engaged in performing a cognitive task, such as learning new words:

- Electromagnetic (ERPs = event-related potentials)
- Optical (EROS = event-related optical signal)
- Three-dimensional (PET = positron emission tomography)
- Magnetic resonance (fMRI = functional magnetic resonance imaging)

If this sounds like alphabet soup, just think about these measures as the x-rays of the twenty-first century. Whereas the x-ray provides a static picture of the interior of the body, these

---

[11] Ibid.

new tools for viewing the brain at work provide dynamic images in three dimensions. It turns out that the brain is more complex, resilient, and adaptive than ever imagined. This is particularly good news for the aging brain that was previously considered too inconsequential to study.

It's hard to know exactly what contributed to the new idea that age is not pathology or that decline is not inevitable. Knowing the exact cause may never be parsed out, whether it was the baby boomers' demand for a robust retirement or science having the means to view a human brain on a computer screen lit up in various colors as the person solved word or number problems for researchers. The fact is that at this very moment in time, being a senior citizen has become just another stage in life, not an inevitable downhill spiral.

In Malcolm Gladwell's bestseller, *Tipping Point,* he shows how various seemingly separate events come together to make a significant, impactful change. The tipping point is like the last link in a chain—hardly significant at the time but completing a cycle that makes a huge difference. Similarly, baby boomers are living at a time when technology-enabled science can literally watch the brain respond in real time. What this means is that it is now becoming possible to see which factors influence health and maximal stimulation for the brain. This is important to us because cognitive enhancement is the outcome, which has signifi-significant impact on the aging brain and its ability to continue to learn and grow.

Another very powerful influence in the last quarter of the twentieth century was an attitudinal shift in the study of aging. The move beyond studying pathology, what's wrong, or what's deteriorated was probably influenced by the wellness movement that gathered momentum in the 70s. It's hard to pinpoint where and how this trend began, but it seems to have been adopted by the flower children of the 60s who were largely countercultural and didn't rely on the traditional medical establishment for health solutions. The first health food stores probably evolved out of the their desire to have an expanded role in self-care and efficacy. Ironically, this same generation of now-aging hippies, and the baby boomers who followed, were the ones who pushed the field of medicine to redefine, or at least expand, the notions surrounding health and pathology in aging.

The shift to the study of health rather than pathology benefits everyone. It is true that some brain-related changes are associated with aging, but that is hardly the whole story. In fact, diseases that arise in this stage of life cause most of the negative changes, but they are definitely not inevitable partners in the aging process. A more valid position is that the brain is a remarkably adaptive and flexible organ that responds to changing needs of the body it serves. That said, it is absolutely critical to use this complex organ well into old age. The use-it-or-lose-it concept is particularly apropos during the Vintage Years.

The Aging Body: How Exercise Stimulates the Brain

The analogy of brain dexterity to physical fitness kept coming up as I did research for this book. Scientists refer to the brain's need for stimulation the way fitness gurus preach muscle toning and flexibility training for the body. Not surprising, the body-mind integration concept is valid, and working on the body actually does facilitate the strengthening of the mind.

A decade ago, the focus of attention was on straightforward physical training programs for post–seventy-year-olds. The results were phenomenal in that older adults with couch-potato habits could make dramatic cardiovascular changes within months and catch up to the most fit of their generation. It wasn't even brain science.

Inactive older folks were instructed in aerobic exercise (walking, using an elliptical trainer, etc.), strength training (using weights and machines), and flexibility (yoga, stretching, etc.) over a six-month period. At the end of that training, the previously unfit had all the benefits of the always-fit older people. Of course, the trick was to continue the practice, because the body, like the brain, benefits and improves with activity—use it or lose it. Dr. Doidge echoes this idea: "Once we reach middle age, we are usually replaying mastered skills. To maintain a brain in good shape, you've got to work as hard as you worked when you learned French vocabulary in high school. People go through decades without that type of training, and the cortex gets dull."[12]

It turns out that what's true for the body is true for the brain. And using the whole brain, the goal-driven part as well as the creative part, may actually be the hallmark of the aging brain.

The Robust Brain

Just within the past decade, specific training programs have been created for both brain flexibility and strength with excellent outcomes. The early work was specific to memory—recall for a list of words, for example—and took place over a brief period of time, like six weeks. The part of the brain that benefits from

---

[12] Ibid.

stimulation of verbal activity responded well. But the approach was specific and not comprehensive.

According to George Rebok, Ph.D., of Johns Hopkins University, whom I heard speak at the Cognitive Aging Summit sponsored by the National Institute on Aging in 2007, "The challenge is to move beyond the standard six-week training program.... I think we need more long-haul, high-impact interventions." To paraphrase Dr. Rebok, if the training is limited in time and scope, the outcomes will be limited as well. But according to Wendy Park, Ph.D., moderator of this conference panel, the research is difficult and time-consuming, so while "behavioral interventions to increase cognitive functioning are definitely the right direction, we just don't know for sure which ones."

As scientists and brain researchers ponder over what kinds of training will have maximal benefits for our brains, we continue to age, and unless we take an active approach to learning, our brains lose ground in the same way that an unexercised body becomes less resilient and strong.

The most powerful statement about continued learning in the Cognitive Aging Summit came from Michael Merzensch, Ph.D., of the Posit Science Corporation, whose comments may be somewhat biased by the fact that his company creates computerized modules to train memory in older adults—perhaps a conflict of interest. Nevertheless, his animated talk suggested that there is a period "in early life which is all about learning and acquisition and development of ability. The brain is a learning machine, and we go into a period in which we are predominantly users of mastered skills and abilities." Here he is describing the brain at a later stage in life where active learning has given way to repetition or even coasting. "We mistake that activity for learning and [it leads to the] disengagement of our learning machine, in a relative sense. It results in the down regulation of the process that guides learning."

His comments resonate with David Kelley's earlier observation of the creatively curious child who succumbs to the more practical demands of education and life—like learning multiplication tables and names of state capitols. These are necessary but not sufficient activities to foster creativity.

When we think about the curiosity of the five-year-old concentrating on learning something, whether it is how to read a word, draw a picture, or put together a puzzle, we can see the brain at work. The same is true for a teen learning to play a new video game or the guitar, or trying to understand the meaning of a book passage. This is a very active learning process that slows and often stops as time goes by unless stimulated in a very engaging and ongoing way. As we know from the last chapter, adulthood can actually lead to stymied brains because of internal and external life requirements that postpone active and creative learning.

What Gets Better With Aging?

The brain's very resilient and flexible nature gives it the capacity to change when we decide to make a change—which often isn't until the demands of earlier life begin to recede. It turns out that this timing is perfect, as the two sides of our brains become more linked and interdependent as we age, amplifying what we are capable of doing, thinking, and seeing. Gene Cohen writes that, "Bilateral brain involvement—can support a more balanced perspective on life that draws on both our logical, analytical powers as well as our nonverbal, intuitive capacities ".[13] While the mature brain, and by that I mean the over-sixty brain, processes more slowly than its young or middle-age counterpart, it is finally situated in a life stage where time is more plentiful and the urgency to get stuff done fast is a thing of the past. If the older brain processes more slowly, it is compensated by its tendency to focus better on individual tasks, having fewer distractions and interferences associated with the complexities of earlier life.

An analogy that comes to mind is the typical twenty, thirty, or forty-something person busy texting, phoning, or computer-surfing all at once while having a conversation and perhaps watching TV. The overuse of technological gadgets, to the point where all brain circuits are occupied, slows down the user's processing speed—independent of age. Older folks' slower but more focused processing speed may not prove to be a disadvantage! So much for decreased processing speed. That argument may be a moot point.

Cohen goes on to say that, "As our brains become more densely wired, they also become less rigidly bifurcated." What this means is that as we age, the right and left sides of the brain begin to work together more than they did before—the logical, rational left side boosting the creative potential of the right side and vice versa. "In most people the left hemisphere specializes in speech, language, and logical reasoning while the right hemisphere handles more intuitive tasks such as face recognition and reading emotional cues ... but this pattern changes as we age."[14]

---

[13] *The Mature* Mind, p.63

[14] Ibid.

The natural evolution of the brain allows older people to use both hemispheres to do a particular task more effectively albeit more slowly. Thinking and feeling are also better integrated than earlier in life. An interesting by-product of this integration is that older men and women are more like each other than they were at any other stage in life since childhood.

The stereotypic perception of men as more logical and women as more emotional problem solvers ceases to have meaning in the Vintage Years in which both genders call upon both sides of the brain more interchangeably. The resulting changes provide equal opportunity for both genders in the development of their inner artist, whether it is as a writer, musician, or visual artist.

Robert Cabeza, a neuroscientist who studies the brainpower of older adults, takes the concept of bilaterality one-step further. He suggests that using both hemispheres allows you to have a more robust approach to problem solving and analogizes this to the way we use our bodies. For example, picking up something heavy with two hands makes more sense and facilitates the process of lifting. Using both sides of your body to do any physical task enhances balance, and so forth. Having the ability to use both sides of your brain as needed facilitates cognitive processing—the work of the brain.

Of course, using both sides of your brain together is technically made possible by simply living longer, but brain training is a conscious choice and requires dedicated action. You might think about it this way: Normal development causes a child's body to mature into an adult body, but maintaining the optimal adult body requires work, as all of us know and to which the industries built around promoting strong, healthy bodies can attest. Strengthen the body as you age, but don't neglect the brain. Exploring the arts is one way to make this happen.

How the Arts Benefit Aging

While interviewing the older artists whose biographies highlight the artistic life in this book, I noticed some significant similarities between them. One striking phenomenon was their ability to focus with laser sharpness while they were engaged in their art. While writing a poem, sculpting, or playing the violin, many described being in an altered state of consciousness, alert and aware but without distraction, in a cocoon where nothing else seemed to matter at that moment.

This kind of focus is described as *flow* by Mihaly Csikszentmihalyi, a psychologist well known for his research on the connection between the state of flow and well-being. He defines this as "concentration so intense that there is no attention left over to think about anything irrelevant or to worry about problems. Self-consciousness disappears, and the sense of time becomes distorted. An activity that produces such experiences is so gratifying that people are willing to do it for its own sake".[15]

Doing something for its own sake is a powerful idea. It encompasses the joy, intensity, and satisfaction that you see in young children looking at the world with fresh eyes, open to new experience and doggedly determined. When it comes to the arts, that kind of exuberance may have to skip over adulthood entirely to find expression—still later in life.

The late-blooming artists I interviewed were well acquainted with the concept of flow, if not with the word itself. In response

---

[15] *Flow: The Psychology of Optimal Experience*, p. 71.

to my question about how many minutes or hours per day they practiced, many could not give me a number. Over and over, I heard that once they entered into a state of absorption with their art, they lost track of time. Clearly, the smell of food coming from the kitchen at dinnertime or the phone ringing would get their attention—but until then, it could be minutes or hours. They weren't always sure. I also heard that pain often ceased to be a focus, even when it was acute. You will meet Judy in Part II. She fell on her knee while walking to her art class but continued to paint, unaware of the swelling and throbbing in her leg until she stood up hours later.

While there is yet no definitive evidence that practicing an art form per se will increase neuronal productivity or match a younger brain's speed, there is evidence that the complexity of cognitive activity through taking on new and challenging projects does enhance functioning. Because taking up an art form is driven by passion, interest, curiosity, sometimes years of waiting, and consciously driven aspiration, focused attention increases in ways or to a degree not likely before.

"Learning triggers the brain to grow," according to Louis Cozolino, psychologist and author of *The Healthy Aging Brain.* "Our activities can have a profound impact on the development of our brains throughout our lives."[16] Unlike researchers in the twentieth century who cared little for the over-forty brain, Dr. Cozolino marvels at the plasticity of the brain, its ability to change, to learn, and to grow new neurons in later life.

Even twenty years ago, the idea of growing new neurons later in life was scientifically laughable. Now, the idea is consid-

---

[16] p. 69

ered mainstream within neuroscience circles. What this means is that growth does indeed continue with nerve cell increase in the brain, albeit not at the same rate as in early and mid adulthood. Nevertheless, the important and more significant changes noted in later adulthood are in the strengthened connections linking nerve cells, referred to as long-term potentiation or LTP.

According to Cozolino, "With age, everyday problem solving and verbal abilities seem to improve."[17] For most of us seniors, this means that our brain, matured over time and having done the typical activities that life over the decades required, is as good or better than ever. A lifetime of learning does count for something, and an older brain is one that has learned much more than its younger counterpart.

Gene Cohen says that learning causes physical changes in the brain and, "an older adult's brain, magnified tremendously, would look distinctly different from a young person's brain." This finding is not surprising and seems logical but may have been misinterpreted by researchers in the twentieth century to mean that different signifies less. Not true! In fact, according to Cohen, "Brain cells in the parts of the brain that an older person has used continuously would look like a dense forest of thickly branched trees, compared with the thinner and less dense forest of a young brain. This neural density is the physical basis for the skills of accomplished older adults."[18]

As suggested before, the aspects of performance that are timed or require speed, as in solving math problems quickly, do

---

[17] p. 67

[18] *The Mature Mind*, p. 5

decline. Fortunately, in the Vintage Years there is little demand for memorizing. The patterns that the brain amassed over half a century provide a solid foundation on which to build. At a practical level, this translates into a brain that is ripe for learning to play an instrument, paint a landscape, or write a short story.

To continue to build connections between neurons and grow more nerve cells requires stimulation: not just any kind of stimulation, but activities that fuel the brain maximally. It turns out that newness or novelty, complexity, and problem solving are very robust tonics for the aging brain. Happily, engaging in the arts strengthens these very qualities in ways that may trump other endeavors.

Creative Aging

Dr. Cohen's research on creativity in later life points to a natural tendency "to reminisce and elaborate stories, either in oral, written, or visual form...part of nature's plan to pass the wisdom of human expression on from one generation to another."[19]

Going back to the beginnings of human time, the role of the elder was to preserve and communicate history and culture to the next generation. There is ample evidence that what we call a natural tendency actually reflects the work of the Vintage brain doing what it was designed to do long ago when the cave wall was the canvas for depicting rituals and showing behaviors necessary for survival.

Evidence in the form of music, created from the first human sounds (grunting, humming, nature sounds) or primitive instruments made of bones and hides, may even predate language.

---

[19] *The Creative Age,* p. 97

While the initial goal was likely to warn others in the tribe about danger and later to document this knowledge for subsequent generations, music, art, and oral narrative survived through the ages, thanks to the elders and to the brain that does not prune what is necessary for survival.

The oral narrative has been part of all cultures and is still a central way of communicating what's important in life in places where the written word is less prevalent. Less than one hundred years ago, right here in the U.S., Native American tribes had very well-developed ways of passing on what was important to remember about life and death through art, music, dance, and storytelling. In the forefront of this process, a spiritual leader, wise one, teacher, or shaman in other cultures—usually an elder—led the way. This practice, it seems, remains the most critical job of the elder: creating and expressing ways to understand the inner and outer worlds.

Even though it was rarely a part of their earlier life plan, elder leaders in most fields have a tendency to communicate what they know during their Vintage Years. It is precisely at this stage in life when the combination of knowledge, experience, and emotional readiness, in conjunction with more available time, finds expression through creative channels.

Think about the memoirs you see displayed at the bookstore or on Amazon.com, most of them penned by gray-haired statespersons, scholars, entrepreneurs, and scientists, as well as everyday people who want to share observations gleaned over a lifetime. We'll meet a few of these artists in later chapters.

Rethinking the Stages in Life

The years during our late fifties to early seventies comprise Phase II of Cohen's four-stage grouping of the second half of life. We focused on the first of these phases in the chapter on Adulthood, picking up where the developmental psychologist Erik Erikson left off at a time when Adulthood was considered the end of the road.

Although none of my interviewees were familiar with Cohen or his definition of Phase II, a time for "liberation, experimentation and innovation . . . and new neuron formation in the information-processing part of the brain associated with a desire for novelty"[20], virtually everyone I interviewed described this process in their own lives and in their own words.

Liberation means openness to taking a risk to do new things, to do the old things differently, or to think differently. It means feeling more secure personally and less worried about making a mistake, or even failing. Remember that learning happens entirely for its own sake and there is much less worry about incompetence and what others think. This particular sentiment resonated without exception in the stories I heard from the budding artists I surveyed.

The liberation phase feels like a second adolescence for most people. Once again, the goal is to push the boundaries and explore one's own uniqueness. For this reason, some of the choices may look extreme to bystanders. This is probably why the term midlife crisis was coined, and yet this stage is rarely a crisis but instead an opportunity to grow outside of the box.

---

[20] p. 52

For example, when Marty, a sculptor whom we will meet in Part II, signed up for a weekend course in Santa Cruz, he had never carved anything before. He was curious and energetically embraced the idea to do something totally different. He was ready to break away from the scientist within who defined his earlier life.

But adolescence isn't always a time of exploration, especially for those who suffered financial or emotional poverty, and the mid-sixties to mid-seventies may be the first point in life where liberation is possible. It's particularly exciting and energizing to finally get the opportunity to freely choose, create, and act. This was true for Betsy, whose teen years were spent being first in her class and following in her parents' academic footsteps. Her diligence got her into a first-rate college and graduate school, but taking artistic risks had to wait until her sixties.

In the next section you will learn more about Betsy and meet the other late-blooming artists who began their work around age sixty, in some cases much later. Their personal stories comprise Part II of *The Vintage Years*.

5 Musicians

A newly released book titled *Guitar Zero* chronicles the experience of thirty-eight-year-old cognitive psychologist, Gary Marcus, who teaches at New York University. He took his sabbatical year to finally learn in earnest how to play the guitar after decades of disappointing starts and stops. His book is about how the brain has enough neuroplasticity to allow an aging, albeit thirty-something person, to learn to play an instrument. He chose to be his own guinea pig and practiced up to six hours a day for eighteen months. To his delight, he learned to play well enough to enjoy his sounds, to play in his own rock band, and even to write music. Do we still have that capacity when we're sixty-five? That's my position and that's what this section is about.

According to Norman Doidge, "Neuroplastic discoveries about adult development are a good reason for the word 'retirement' to itself be retired. We may be happiest if we work our brains as hard as ever—doing something we love."[21] This is good news for Vintage Years folks.

Finding your inner musician six decades into life was unimaginable until the twenty-first century. Prior to that time, a talk with any group of serious musicians or musicologists would yield consensus about the need to begin study as a child, a very young child for that matter. Thankfully, scientific thinking is changing. Only recently have I gotten a glimpse into what a sixty-year-old set of hands and eyes, combined with heart and mind, can produce in the way of music. The stories of the late-blooming musicians who graciously allowed me to interview them follow.

---

[21] Interview with Allan Gregg on *Science Friday*; TV Ontario, 10/25/10

1 John: Piano Student

John intrigued me from the moment a friend told me about him. At eighty-eight, he had been playing the piano for eight years. After introducing my project and myself by e-mail, I encountered a hard sell convincing him to meet with me. About his playing, he energetically quipped, "Approaching eighty-eight, I seem qualified per your age brackets, but from the artistic aspect, I don't believe I can be useful to you. There isn't anything I do that involves creative expression. At age eighty, I made the mistake of buying a piano and taking the very first music lesson of my life. The only positive thing I can say about the experience is that my teacher has not yet committed suicide!"

This was quite an introduction, and his disclaimer only made me more interested in meeting the man. I approached him by e-mail again, and though he seemed to not agree with me about the usefulness of the meeting, he agreed to do it anyway if I thought it worthwhile. I was prepared to meet him at his home in San Francisco and possibly see him at his piano, but he suggested the Lake Merced Golf Club where he is an active member and which was closer for me. I suspected that part of the decision was based on his reticence to demonstrate his piano skills if he were stuck with me in the very room where his piano resides.

In preparation for the interview, I tried to learn more about John from an online search. All I could find was a picture of him and his wife, Marie, taken a year before at a party for the president of the San Francisco Opera. The stately couple in formal wear peering at me through the computer image served only to help me identify them at the club. This picture, while a reference point, made me feel a little uneasy as I found their formal attire translating into a formal, prim, and proper meeting in my mind. It was anything but.

John looked preppy in a brightly colored V-neck sweater under a light windbreaker. Although it was late July, the San Francisco Bay coastal morning fog kept the day cool. Marie had come along to listen to the interview and to chime in with her perception of John from time to time. After a strong handshake, he seated me next to him in the club restaurant and began to talk comfortably and easily about the eighty years that preceded his piano playing.

No one's life is easy to summarize in an hour, but I could see that his would be especially difficult. If I could identify a theme going though his life, it was his perception that much happened to him by accident or happenstance. Downplaying his accomplishments, including his piano foray, was not so much a put-down as it was a way of explaining a life full of surprising twists and turns built on his curious nature.

Growing up near San Jose, the area now known as Silicon Valley where computer chips are grown instead of the fruits and vegetables of fifty years ago, John entered college only to flunk out by the next year. It was 1942, and he joined the Navy where he spent the next four years. Following the war, he applied for readmission to his former college, but they didn't think him worthy of another chance. Undaunted, he went to another local college where he finished out his years as a straight-A student.

According to John, he wound up in graduate school in an unexpected way, but I think it was because of the intense curiosity I observed in him during our interview. Long story short, he emerged with a Ph.D. in organic chemistry. Again and again, he pointed to luck and happenstance directing him forward, not seeing his strong role in making things happen for himself. "My entire career has been an accident—a good one, but an accident. Strange events happened." While not being cryptic, he felt a need to explain and make sense of the irregular path. Embracing the piano was one of those strange happenings.

A series of adventuresome career choices let John follow his instincts and passion, first abroad in Switzerland and then in Mexico where his chemistry background took him, and later in San Francisco where he and Marie retired. Fast-forward to his mid-seventies, and John was now a loyal patron of the arts: opera, symphony, and ballet.

As sponsors of young performing artists, the couple had ample opportunity to sample some of the best classical music available. It was when they moved into a large apartment with a generous-sized living room "with room for a piano, and a perfect spot for a piano" that the idea of owning a piano was born. This idea was presented to me as another happenstance or chance situation.

When asked if the piano was viewed as a piece of furniture, John was quick to say that it wasn't, which suggested that there was some plan, however loosely construed, to use it for the production of music. It turns out that the choice was inspired following years of hosting young musicians at his home, one of whom was a pianist. "When I thought to buy a piano, I didn't know anything about pianos, but Laura (years later an established piano teacher) does. So she came and helped us buy a piano, and after that the question became, 'So who's going to give me lessons?' And Laura helped find a teacher—who has suffered with me these eight years." At eighty, John began his lessons. "I was always interested in the piano. I just didn't think I would ever do anything with it. It just never occurred to me until we moved to San Francisco and had all the time and space for a piano."

As I tried to drill down to John's motivation and goals in taking on the study of music at eighty, he volunteered, "I'm not joking, I'm being serious when I tell you this. I recognized that I might never learn how to play the piano, but at least I might be able to read the squiggles on the page, and that would already be something of an achievement." That was exactly what he said to his wife years earlier, who validated his words by nodding in agreement with an affectionate smile and clear support of his endeavor.

"Right now I've been working for about five months on a Chopin prelude. I don't anticipate that I will ever be able to play it." I reminded him that he was indeed playing it, so he further clarified his meaning. "Oh, well, I can't play it without error. It's a huge problem for me. I never dreamed that reading music would be so damned difficult." I think that John forgot his original intent, and like most adults with sophisticated listening skills, overlooked the accomplishment and enjoyment of translating the squiggles on the page into sound.

His irritability at the slowness of his progress became the focus of conversation. It's taken him three months to get to page three of the written music, and he still finds reading music a great challenge, insisting that the whole process is difficult and playing in front of others is out of the question. He shared in hushed tones, as if telling a secret, that he will stop playing if anyone enters the room, even the lady who cleans his apartment. The only exception is Marie, who looks at him lovingly across the table. There's no doubt that she is proud of his playing, enjoys his involvement with the piano, and doesn't have a judging bone in her body.

While John is unsure why he continues to play, he does on a fairly regular basis. Almost every day finds him at the piano for a brief practice, sometimes only ten minutes, often twenty, but rarely longer. He does admit, although almost grudgingly, that he has much more understanding of how music works, and this increases his appreciation of the music he loves.

He beamed as he excitedly told the story of a piece of classical music: "The fourth movement of Mahler's Ninth Symphony, with Leonard Bernstein conducting the Viennese Philharmonic, in the first four minutes of music you can compare that to ..." He launched into a very sophisticated comparison with another orchestra's interpretation of the same music; he had listened to both on his computer. "The first interpretation was so incredibly moving," he recalls, almost swaying to the music in his head and visibly filled with emotion. He was able to appreciate the subtle style differences and realized that he had a preference. Years spent playing the piano and reading music, albeit slowly and painstakingly, finely tuned his preferences and increased his sophistication as a listener. This is why he hasn't quit playing, he says.

One thread that runs though many interviews is the relationship that comes about between the artist and a new friend built completely around their shared art. In John's case, it is an eight-year relationship with his piano teacher that is personally very meaningful and more than balances his frustration.

When asked about his health, he replied it was excellent. He could not answer the question about how his art affected his health. Marie suggested that his mental health was much better, and he agreed with her perception. As we were closing our meeting, he commented that mental health was part of health, so maybe his health was positively affected by his art after all. Then he excused himself and dashed off to play some golf.

2   Charmion: Viola da Gamba

Charmion just moved to a small coastal town known as Soquel near Santa Cruz, California. The most recent of her many moves around the U.S., this one followed the death of her second husband a few years ago. At eighty-one, she's finally set down roots not far from her daughter. I was hoping to learn how she chose to study the viola da Gamba—an exotic, ancient instrument resembling a cello in appearance but having a very different heritage.

After changing our meeting time because of the new tai chi class she wanted to take, we met at the home she shares with her dog, Electra. Charmion, whose name comes from a Shakespearean character associated with poisoning Queen Cleopatra, is as fascinating as her name.

Sitting across from me at her dining room table, drinking half-caf lattes produced by her new espresso machine, she began to offer her life story before I could get my recorder started. "I decided that I needed to find out if I was creative," she announced, jumping right into the near end of her story. "I prefer to think about myself as a Renaissance woman," she continued, describing a situation when she was about seventy years old and curious about who she was separate from the roles she assumed and those imposed on her throughout her earlier life. This was the first point in her life that she stopped to take inventory. Her husband had just retired and the world opened up in ways not visible before. Her experience seemed typical for Vintage Years men and women, though her life was not the least bit mainstream.

Her remarkable story began in Detroit, the daughter of a very successful real estate developer and young stay-at-home mother. When Charmion was only a year old, her world was turned upside down when her father shot her mother and then killed himself. Although her mother survived, the family wealth was distributed to her father's family of origin, leaving her and her mother penniless.

A highly resourceful woman, Charmion's mother managed to find a job and to make ends meet. But after four years, she yearned for a new start away from the lingering stigma of her husband's rampage. In 1934, she loaded up the car and drove across the country to California, the land of opportunity. She was always able to find some kind of work in the growing movie industry that defined Los Angeles at that time.

This strong-willed, bright, educated, ambitious mother decided that Charmion could become a little Shirley Temple and set about making that happen by providing her with voice and dance lessons. Although reluctant and not sharing her mother's vision, Charmion went along with her forceful mother's plan. She confided to me that she continued to do what Mother wanted until she was eighteen. But the California plan was short lived.

In 1942, in the midst of World War II when Charmion was twelve, Mother joined the army, and Charmion was sent to boarding school in Michigan. Charmion's summers were spent in camp, and she had no home or permanent address. Fortunately for Charmion, she had a good voice, good survival skills, and a superior intellect. Before finishing high school, she had attended more than ten different schools.

Reaching the rank of captain, her mother returned to Michigan, set up a household, and once again influenced her daughter's decisions. Now the plan was to move to New York where, at eighteen, Charmion was pushed toward more serious voice lessons. "It never crossed my mind that what I wanted might be different than what my mother wanted. Momentarily, I thought I wanted to be a veterinarian because I loved horses like a lot of young girls do, but I mentioned it to my mother and she said, 'Oh, no, that's ridiculous—you're going to be a singer.' If I had any other thoughts, they were gone."

Keeping her day job as a secretary, Charmion was able to get some professional work singing in a church choir. But at nineteen: "I joined the army to get away from my very domineering mother. After one day, I realized I'd made the biggest mistake of my life." Her military career was short lived. After slightly more than two years, she was discharged. That seemed like an extremely short commitment to me, so I must have looked perplexed. Charmion said, "I got pregnant. That got me out."

She returned to California and went to UCLA under the G.I. Bill, but life got in the way again. A brief marriage and another child cut short her education. Start, stop, start again; Charmion's life continued to unfold in a choppy fashion, but her singing continued and she recalled, "I had an opportunity to tour with Roger Wagner's choir, big in the 50s, and I left my husband and two kids—I walked off and went touring. After a couple of years, I divorced my husband." She volunteered a bit sheepishly that her growing-up years didn't provide her with a traditional married-with-children model of life. "But, I was a soloist with the Los Angeles Philharmonic Orchestra," she quickly added, perhaps to justify her decision to keep singing as her primary objective.

Clearly, Charmion's unusual life is almost impossible to summarize in a few pages, and like you, I was getting anxious to learn about her post-retirement artistry, fully aware that our time together was ticking away. Attempting to tie together some threads from her history, I learned that she quit touring to give her school-aged kids more stability, and after her kids finished high school, she returned to UCLA, completing a bachelor's degree in Analysis and Conservation of Ecosystems, a science curriculum that was very challenging and a long way off from music!

"I got a master's degree in Biological Geography, and that was so much fun, I decided to get a doctorate." Once again, Charmion changed direction just as she was getting ready to write her dissertation. "By now, I was in my early sixties and it seemed ridiculous. So, I retired out of college," she laughed heartily. I agreed that she's done everything in novel ways.

"I've been a rather unproductive person," she lamented, which prompted me to give a little talk about cultural values and life stages. Productivity is a concept that is highly valued in many cultures of the Western world, and greatly inflated in importance. We tend to measure our worth by it, but it's not the only yardstick. It's a narrow and maybe a shallow way to view ourselves. In our twenties, thirties, and forties, along with the need to make a living, we want to do something to make a mark on the world. But by sixty, our goals are different, driven at this stage of life by passion, meaning, and what feels authentic.

Charmion nodded slowly as if she was still digesting my mini-lecture but then launched into a somewhat unrelated subject. "At seventy-one, I decided that I was far too left-brained. I started to wonder if I had any right brain at all and decided to investigate that. From my perspective, singers are basically not creative people. I think they could be, but I think they are performers of somebody else's creativity. Others might argue with this, but I was not a creative singer; I did whatever the composer and conductor wanted."

Coming full circle to the beginning of the interview, Charmion reasserted her concern that she might not be very creative: "I took a couple of courses in poetry writing at the junior college." With no background or training, and "limited exposure in high school writing classes, I found that I really enjoyed writing. There's something cathartic in it. I got into a group that met periodically and discussed and read poetry to each other." Since her move to northern California, she admits to doing less with writing than she would like, but she satisfied her curiosity about her own creativity.

Charmion's creativity quest led her in new directions to new adventures. First came the challenge of teaching herself how to play the recorder, a humble flute-like instrument popular in the sixteenth and seventeenth centuries and more recently in the curricula of well-endowed elementary school music programs. "I decided I wanted to learn how to play a musical instrument, and the recorder is a very simple instrument. After I got beyond the basics, I got a teacher." I wondered how much time she devoted to learning the recorder. Four hours a week, was her response, roughly a half-hour at a time, but with no regular schedule, just the commitment to herself that she would do it. She's very determined and good with follow-through, clearly part of her na-

nature but also a skill she learned for managing her early chaotic life.

Charmion segued to talking about the viola da Gamba, her current passion. She doesn't recommend it as a starter instrument and finds its six strings and an unusual bow hold very difficult. She emphatically said that it is even more difficult than the cello, which I can't even imagine! Taking notice of my puzzled expression—why someone would choose such a demanding hobby—she quickly added that she adores early music, medieval and Renaissance, maybe from her days singing church music in a choir. "I enjoy the challenge. I like the sound."

A friend suggested the viola da Gamba. "I think I should kill her for that. It's very hard," she chuckled, "but I enjoy the challenge. I like challenges. Once in a while, I make a great sound, and it's beautiful when I do." Charmion practices everyday from 6:00–7:00 a.m. It's the first thing she does after waking, and some days she makes time for an additional hour of practice. She is quite serious about getting better, although at this moment, she won't play for anyone but her teacher. I tried to get her to play a few notes when I snapped a posed picture of her holding the viola da Gamba. She politely refused!

Referring to her playing, she said, "Everything I've ever read and everything I've experienced tells me that this is conducive to keeping me mentally sharp. There's also a physical coordination required, particularly on an instrument like the da Gamba—physical and yet not terribly demanding of old bodies." I very much agree that the fine arts require a certain amount of physicality in addition to the mental workout.

Regarding the unwieldy, cello-like size of her instrument, I laughed and remarked that just lugging it around required some strength and coordination. Coming again full circle to her new tai chi class, Charmion suggested that her motivation for it is about balance, helpful for the da Gamba and definitely useful for post-sixty physiques.

Realizing that we were out of time, and quickly trying to summarize, I asked for any advice she might have for a new retiree or anyone past sixty who is looking for a new and meaningful pastime. She reflected for just a second and then emphatically said to "use your own style to guide you. If you are an introvert, then maybe read books and do Internet searches until something resonates with your interests. If you are an extravert, then your starting point might be some community classes or workshops." This distinction of personality style is useful and echoes what I've heard from others.

As she walked me to the door, I realized that at eighty-one, Charmion is as alert and agile as any middle-aged person I can think of. I wonder, is eighty-one the new fifty-five or sixty?

3 Don: Fiddler and Violin Maker

I'm a city girl, so the trip winding through the mountains toward the Livermore valley in north-central California, culminating on a one-lane road, seemed treacherous on this drizzly, fog-enshrouded day. When I finally arrived at the compound near the peak of Mt. Diablo, I was shaken but relieved as Don greeted me in his driveway.

Wearing jeans, a workman's shirt, and a broad-rimmed hat resembling the kind that cowboys wear, he was the picture of outdoor ruggedness and health. He ushered me inside through the sunroom on the front of his sprawling house, built on a fourteen-acre hillside, replete with two donkeys that keep the grass short, which helps to prevent summer forest fires. I knew that goats were kept by farmers to trim large meadows but hadn't realized that donkeys do the same kind of work. Don said that he used to keep a herd of cattle as well, but it got too complicated since he isn't really a farmer or rancher.

Don got his college degree in Physics in 1956 and spent his career as a physicist working for a long stretch at the Lawrence Livermore National Laboratory, a federal facility that studies the effect of atomic explosions. He focused on the environmental impact of such explosions on soil. Interest in the environment led him to build a solar house, heated entirely by the sunroom that wraps around half of his house. He explained that a windmill erected on his land previously generated all of their electricity. In a terrible storm a while back, the tall structure with its ten-foot blades collapsed. Now they are back on the grid!

With a myriad of other interests tugging on his time, Don retired at age fifty-six. Physics is still a fascination for him, but his lifelong love of wood, bronze, and marble sculpting, as well as old car restoration, demanded more attention than a working person could reasonably provide. "I wanted the time more than the money," he said—a reasonable trade off for someone who lives lightly on the land in a very remote, rural area in a home he built himself.

A few years after retirement, Don and his wife visited his sister who lived in Nova Scotia. She played the fiddle, basically a violin used to play folk music—to be precise in her case, Scottish folk tunes that came down through the ages. When Don left, she gave him one of several fiddles she played and told him to fool around with it when he got home. Don was naturally curious, so he took it with no thought as to what he would do with it. Little did he know at that time that this would become a burning passion that would shape his next fifteen years. Don was sixty-three at the time.

Don is currently seventy-eight, and here's a snapshot of his current life: He wakes at 5:00 a.m. and plays the fiddle until 7:00 a.m. "I keep a pretty rigid schedule for playing. If I didn't get it done in the morning, I would never stop later to do it when I get busy with other things. My wife sleeps until 7:00 a.m., and I'm done practicing by the time she wakes up, which works out very nicely for me," he says with a smile, implying that his sound might be annoying. I heard him play later and it was anything but.

"I sometimes wonder, why in the world would a seventy-eight-year-old man keep trying to play the fiddle and keep taking lessons now and then, but I think, at my age, it's to keep my fingers and my hand moving. I've memorized about three hundred tunes. That's a good feeling. It's also very satisfying to say that last year I couldn't do that." As he beamed with pride, he answered his own question.

In the course of our discussion, Don told me that he played clarinet in high school and college and learned to read music, "which is now helpful to me in my current study of classical violin music—you know, Hayden, Mozart, Beethoven, and a host of other composers from the Baroque period." This was a surprise to me, and I realized that his foray into music did not happen late in life, which was one criterion necessary for inclusion in my study. I decided to tell you his story anyway, because while the clarinet is indeed a musical instrument, and Don is no newcomer to understanding music, it isn't a stringed instrument and he was a beginner at sixty-three.

My theory is that it is possible in the Vintage Years to learn to play a musical instrument and that while there may be some benefit derived from earlier music training, you must still walk the walk, which means practicing, practicing, practicing and learning a whole new set of skills, like using a bow and holding your left note-playing hand at the correct angle.

When there was a lull in the dialogue, I found myself giving a mini lecture about what allows the brain to function optimally at later stages in life. Novelty, complexity, and problem solving are so much a part of learning to play an instrument, as they are with other art forms, I noted. I hoped Don would comment on whether these factors were relevant to him. "If there is a part of a piece that I'm trying to play, and it doesn't matter whether it's classical music or fiddle tunes, you get to a place where you say that is just impossible, and so you just work on it, and work on it, and in a month it's possible," he says laughing. "There's a piece I'm actually working on that's very challenging; it's called 'Madame Neruta.' Just in the past few days, I've got that almost mastered." He spoke about the novelty and complexity of the piece and the excitement of conquering it. I suggested that his brain was getting a good workout, and we both laughed at the visual image this created.

It turns out that his favorite musical experience is playing in the yearly Scottish Fiddlers' concert with as many as one hundred and ten musicians on the stage, playing tunes from memory—no music stands or sheet music allowed—though some participants tape their music to the chair in front of them, a little cheat sheet, I guess. He doesn't enjoy the monthly fiddler meetings as the best players tend to drive the pace, which is somewhat competitive and too fast for Don. Most of the time, he is content to play for himself.

Recently, he's been diagnosed with a vision problem that makes it more challenging to read music, but Don has been determined to find ways to accommodate his playing. In this case, he uses more intense light shining directly at the page. Also, he has some arthritis in his left thumb, but it isn't noticeable while he's playing or building violins.

"I have a friend, and when he retired all he wanted to do was play golf, and pretty soon he got tired of it. With golf, it's a whole lot of money going out the door continuously and you've got nothing to show for it except maybe a trophy." He reminded me of his lifelong hobby of sculpting and later showed me the first piece he created when he was a cub scout: a small wood carving of a horse, still displayed on a book shelf we passed on the way to his violin-making studio. "I get my kicks out of doing something where there is a final product," he said, summing up his choices of hobbies including violin playing and instrument crafting.

Before I left, Don showed me some of the violins he's made and played a Scottish tune on his fifteenth iteration—his best, according to him and beautifully constructed, in my opinion. Though way beyond my ability to understand the technique of violin construction, he patiently pointed out the process, forms, and tools required. I felt like I was transported back in time to a seventeenth-century Italian music master's studio with recently completed instruments hanging from the rafters on hooks. Of course, it made sense. Don is truly a Renaissance man!

4 Barbara: African Drummer

At one time, Barbara was a dance therapist. That was long ago, but her love of dance continued after she changed professions. In truth, studying modern dance in college met some of the two-year physical education requirement at the time. "I think what I found was that I was most focused when I was dancing, whereas when I was in a lecture class, my mind would be wandering. But in the dance class, I was more attentive. It was challenging and I liked the physical release."

The pleasure she derived from moving her body initially led to training as a dance therapist after college. Some time later, when she attended an African dance class recommended by a friend, she became hooked. "I loved it because this kind of movement was easier for my body; it came more naturally. And the rhythm—we had live drummers in the class. There was an old Haitian guy teaching this class. I thought, 'Oh, the drumming looks so cool. Someday, I'm going to do that, but it took me a while to get there," she laughed because it actually took decades.

Barbara and I are friends; and her immersion in drumming made me curious about her attraction to this unconventional musical genre. Willing to tell her story and share her passion, she invited me to her home for a first-hand look and demonstration. The colors in her home were earth tones, soothing to me and characteristic of Barbara's style, but a contrast to the drummer in her who played with abandon. She joined me on the family room couch, comfortably stretched out across from me, graceful as a dancer. The youthful way she carried herself suggested a woman younger than her sixty-two years.

Growing up on Long Island in New York, in the 1960s did not particularly inspire her current musical interests. Neither did her parents who had traditional taste in music and little inclination to play musical instruments. But they did buy Barbara a very simple chord organ when she was a child. "I wouldn't say that I loved it, but sometimes I would get into it and sort of get lost in it. Then the volume would go up and my mother would yell, 'Turn that thing down!'" Barbara laughed at the long-ago memory.

The years passed. Moving to California with her college-sweetheart husband, raising a daughter, and pursuing a new profession kept her busy in the ways that the decades-long Adulthood phase of life does for most of us. Periodically, she would recall the African dance and drumming she loved while attending a group performance at a local event. "Someday, I'm going to do that," she thought, but it would go on the back burner for many years.

West African traditional dance piqued Barbara's interest, and she began taking classes at a local community center where, like in classes she remembered from years before, drummers played the rhythm. Once a week, she danced barefoot with a brightly-flowered and geometric-patterned sash around her waist, which transported her far beyond her home in northern California. Over time, her fascination with the rhythmic tempo and beat of the drums led her to playing drums in the style of central Africa.

"A friend told me about this drumming class. It was very focusing and when we got into the groove of the rhythm, I really liked it. I've stuck with it for nine years." Her teacher had studied with and became very close to Babatunde Olatunji, the Nigerian drummer whose 1959 album, *Drums of Passion,* introduced a mass public in the U.S. to the exotic and vivid sounds of African drums. His name resonated from my own young adult years and the long hours spent listening to music on the stereo. "She transmitted a lot of his technique for learning drumming," Barbara recalled about her teacher. "And from there, I heard about another class."

Considering that Barbara continues to work, I wondered how she integrates the drumming into her busy life. "Now, most of the time that I spend practicing is at the Saturday class I take every week for three to four hours. At different times, I've spent more evening time doing it. Right now, maybe once a week, I kind of practice. When we do some performing, that takes extra time for rehearsal." She usually practices when her husband is out, "So I don't have to worry about disturbing him," she giggled, perhaps remembering her mother's reaction to the loud organ playing a half century before.

Over the last five years, Barbara has become increasingly serious about her playing and now enjoys occasional paid gigs with a makeshift group of musicians. Maybe the ease she feels is one of the hallmarks of being on the other side of sixty.

We talked about what the drums do for her. "If I'm really stressed, the repetitive part of the rhythm can be soothing in itself. It's very relaxing and I'm doing something kind of physical." Barbara talked about the challenge of experimenting with how different aspects of a drumming piece fit together. "There's something about the drums and the bass-grounding quality of drumming that helps me feel more rooted or grounded, centered, and can stimulate me to move as I'm playing—the integration of body and mind." "Spoken like a psychologist," I thought, which she is. But mostly, she plays for fun.

Asking my standard question about the relationship between practicing an art form and general health, Barbara offered her insight. "I think it's irrelevant to my overall health, because I've gotten older in the past nine years, so I have more aches and pains." She laughs as she states the obvious, but then goes on, "But I think my mental health is better. In general, the experience of drumming with other people is pretty energizing, and I think there's something healing about the rhythms themselves, how they are used in African culture."

While explaining the meaning of drumming in Africa, she demonstrated the djembe, a drum of the Mandinka people. It is made from a single piece of wood, carved into the shape of a goblet and hollow throughout. Goatskin, pulled tight on top, is fastened with a natural material: oddly, American rope works best. The djembe appeared timeless, with a deep patina and a shell made of local woods—Barbara wasn't sure what kind— from Mali. Drums have different rhythms associated with different purposes. For example, the rhythm of the djembe might be performed in the evening for most celebrations; during a full moon; for spring, summer, and winter harvesting time; or for weddings, baptisms, and honoring of mothers.

Barbara played barehanded, chopping at the drum sideways with the meat of her hand and alternating that gesture with the smacking sound of her hands falling flat on the drumhead for a different effect. Her playing mesmerized me—the rhythm was haunting and tribal, and I was transported back in time to our primordial ancestors sitting around the evening fire. Barbara swayed to the music and her hands seemed to take on increased powerfulness. I know she wasn't in a trance, because she spoke from time to time, but the far-off look on her face made it seem that way.

Later, she summed up her feelings. "When the rhythm is working right, it's almost like a high. With these particular rhythms, sometimes they're so complex and interwoven—called polyrhythms—that you get this kind of perceptual shift where things that were sounding one way sound a different way." I suggested that it might be like looking through a kaleidoscope or creating a psychedelic experience. We both laugh at the flower-child musical image of the 70s.

I commented that drum rhythm has been a part of life on the earth as far back as humanoids go. It's part of my premise in writing this book that music serves a very basic purpose in culture, both in telling stories and by stimulating emotion, thereby triggering the release of endorphins that have a positive effect on health and mental health. "There's something about rhythm itself that I respond to a lot," Barbara added.

Regarding any future plans, like possible retirement, Barbara's not sure. But if she had more time: "I would take some other music classes, I would do more and different kinds of percussions, I think I might study middle-eastern drumming."

As we parted, I thought, "Who would guess that a conservatively dressed, sixty-something white woman spent a month last year in the northwest African country of Gambia, studying west African drum technique with a chap from Guinea in a small village?" Barbara beamed as she told her story about her very interesting life and the many people, so different from herself, whom she's met along the way.

She explained that drum music naturally expanded her life to experiences and people she would otherwise never encounter. "Music has introduced me to people who are younger and who are from different ethnic backgrounds, different socio-economic statuses, different professions, and different perspectives. Whereas therapists tend to be introspective, I've met people who just want to have fun." Here her voice and tone elevated for emphasis, as she gestured flamboyantly with her arm, laughing as she added, "And drink and party!"

These days, Barbara's idea of a vacation means "going to music camp in different parts of the country and meeting a lot of people who have alternative lifestyles. It has opened a bunch of doors. I've gotten used to performing a little and feel less shy about that. I've gotten more comfortable." In fact, it was her increased confidence with new situations that allowed her to take that extraordinary trip to Africa.

6 Visual Artists

It's easy to visualize an elder sitting alongside a charming landscape, portable easel in arm's reach, with an umbrella attached at the frame to block direct sun. This image resonates with what many of us imagine when we think of the Vintage Years. It turned out that a good many of the people in my study fit into the visual arts category, too many, in fact, to record all of their stories in this book.

One story that didn't make it into the book is my mother's; she seems to have had an imaginary love affair with the French Impressionist artist, Toulouse-Lautrec. This didn't come about until her mid fifties when she was a widow with an empty nest and an artist's eye. Finally, she had the time to try her hand as a conduit of her creativity. Untrained and unconcerned about her lack of formal knowledge, she used every medium I can imagine a hand executing: charcoal, watercolors, tempera, and oils. She applied these to all manner of objects from brown paper bags to canvases.

Mom was prolific and worked very quickly, having little patience for editing. To everyone's surprise, she even had a few shows and sold some paintings. My home is filled with her work, although legacy was not important to her. Happiest while painting in the French Impressionist style, I think she would really have preferred to live in Paris in the mid-nineteenth century. Her sketching, drawing, and painting career ended in her late seventies when she died suddenly.

The eleven stories that follow represent the tremendously varied art forms of women and men who, like my mother, saved their artistry for their Vintage Years.

1 Henry: Woodcarver and Organist

Henry, a tall attractive man dressed youthfully in light colored khakis and a crisp plaid shirt, met me at the door with his walker. At ninety-six, he lives alone and independently with a full life and a busy calendar. His punctual style is marked and reinforced by the numerous clocks that chimed throughout his home only slightly apart on the hour and half hour. I knew in advance not to be late, as Henry does not like to be kept waiting, which made two of us.

I let him know that I would take only an hour of his time but had a feeling after our first words were exchanged that two hours might be a better target. Sharpened by extraordinary recall and a penchant for detail, his stories were captivating. We sat across from each other on matching sofas surrounded by reminders of his long and satisfying life. Pictures of his children, grandchildren, and great grandchildren sat on tables, bookshelves, and walls.

The tastefully decorated bungalow in an active senior residential community in central New Jersey has been his home since retirement at sixty-eight. It was in the community center, the central hub of Concordia, where he first saw an art show nearly thirty years ago that changed his life. Walking through the exhibit, he excitedly commented to his wife at his side, "This is what I like. I want to do this," referring to a large, detailed woodcarving. And so began his long Vintage-Years career as a woodcarver. It was particularly ironic, since carving with a knife was a learned and well-practiced skill in his previous career as a butcher.

Henry was the only son of a meat supplier in Manhattan, New York. At seventeen, Henry entered the business after high school graduation to help his dad and also to find a role in the business for himself. In those days, beef, lamb, and other meats arrived in quarters to be further butchered into various cuts and delivered to businesses. Henry got his start at the proverbial butcher's block, a huge piece of wood, four feet high and wide on which quarters became cuts of meat by Henry's cleaver and butchering knife. With a far away look in his eyes, he described the process of becoming a butcher but hadn't thought until today that his skill with a knife would come in so handy more than fifty years later.

Actually, the story goes back even further. Henry reminded me that kids back in his youth didn't have the ready-made toys of today. To entertain himself, he made things, and some required a knife. He specifically recalled as a seven-year-old making a tank out of a wooden spool used to hold thread. "They are made of plastic these days," he asserted. Detailing the process, he described carving little nicks in the spool with a knife and wrapping the toy with rubber bands so that it rolled along and jumped over obstacles. I couldn't exactly picture it, but grinning, he had a faraway look as he remembered, and the memory foretold his emerging creativity.

While the artist in him would take decades to surface, the meat business benefited from his imagination. Henry's father supported his son's ideas, such as putting an external horn on the delivery truck that resembled a bicycle horn with a long tube ending in a bulb that, when squeezed, would produce a loud honk, or painting the outside of the truck with a sprayer designed for insecticides, creating a splotchy but interesting design. Later, his decision to build an elevator to transport heavy pallets of beef from the meat plant's first-floor delivery to the second-floor cutting room was innovative and readily supported by his dad, who recognized that Henry had talent in aspects of the meat business besides butchering.

For many years, Henry called on hospitals, colleges, and other institutions in Manhattan to increase the wholesale part of the business. Between the work, raising a family, and attending to his wife, the years passed. When asked about other ways he spent his time, he said, "I worked long hours. I got started at 5:00 a.m. and whatever time was left was spent with the kids and their interests." Typical, I thought, of that stage in life. No time for the expression of his creativity, except through his work and vicariously through his children's pursuits.

In the midst of his long career, he designed a branding iron with the family logo: a letter *L* within a triangle that was constructed by a farrier, or horseshoe maker. The brand identified the steaks, bacon, and other products the family sold to restaurants. Little did he know that his logo would become his signature on the sculptures, woodcarvings, and 3-D art that his creativity expressed in his Vintage Years.

I listened intently as Henry tried to compress his long and interesting life. His ability to communicate seemed remarkable. I realized with disappointment that even I had stereotypes about age; I hardly expected a ninety-six-year-old to keep up with me and even initiate conversation about life, meaning, problem solving, trying new things, world history, and travel.

He had a tendency to elaborate on the wonderful details of his art work—a woodcarving of the Taj Mahal, for example, complete with a carved subtitle written in an Indian dialect and the accompanying story about how his dental hygienist of Indian descent had written *Taj Mahal* for him to copy and inscribe on his art work so it would seem more authentic.

Acutely aware of the clocks ticking around me and my promise to take only an hour of his time, I wondered if I could complete our interview without steering Henry in a way that would seem rude, and yet there was so much more to hear and see. With some discomfort, I guided him back to the topic of woodcarving, the first of his art forms that he tackled after seeing that fateful art show when he was sixty-eight.

Woodcarving requires some strength as well as dexterity, and until recently, Henry could lift and drag huge hunks of wood. He took me out to his garage where he asked me to lift a block of his last, but never completed, work sitting alongside a sketch of it. It must have weighed thirty pounds and measured about the size of a sheet of letter paper, but it was at least two inches thick. At sixty-eight, seventy-eight, or even eighty-eight, woodcarving had still been manageable. But not at ninety-six, Henry explained without much sadness. I paused, waiting for some acknowledgement of sorrow or regret about his diminished strength, but none came. Instead, he launched into discussing his newest projects in the genre of 3-D art.

In the first years, the woodcarving classes he diligently attended each week at the community club filled his time. Henry soon added sculpture to his repertoire of skills, preferring to work in three dimensions. His life-size busts of two of his grandchildren sat on pillars in his living room, looking at him with appreciation and reminding him that the butcher knife, which he learned to carve with some eighty years ago, was metaphorically put to good use in the present.

When queried about how he spends his time these days, he referred to the one art class that he takes each week and then reminded me that at ninety-six, "I rest a lot. I need a lot of rest. I get tired easily." I kept forgetting that Henry moves slowly with the help of a walker, but he does get around and still drives. Just as I thought we might be done, and that his message about being tired was directed at me, he chimed in, "I also play music. I play the organ." I hadn't heard about his musical interest until this moment, and my ears perked up. Self-taught, he suggested that playing the organ was another skill he developed after retirement. He laughed as he told me about his one musical composition called, "Meats are Fine," complete with lyrics.

He pulled out a composition pad, the kind musicians use with lines to separate the notes, and on its yellowing pages was the song he wrote at seventy-five. Better yet, he energetically moved across the room to his organ, a modern computer-assisted instrument with all the bells and whistles. He played several pieces to demonstrate the versatility of his organ, like a salesperson eager to close a sale. Then Henry played "Meats are Fine" in honor of his lengthy career and in tribute to his father's meat business. We both had a good laugh and I greatly enjoyed his playfulness.

Although he composed only one song, he described how he modifies this piece and others with flourishes: a different beat, a new accent, a modified chord. "Sometimes when I'm having dinner, I get an idea and I run over to the organ to try it out. I get into playing and totally forget about dinner. I just get lost in it." I interjected that what he described is called *flow*, the process of being so involved in what you do that it's easy to lose track of time and the experience feels invigorating, pleasurable, even restorative. His word to sum up the experience is *relaxing*.

Henry credits his daily physical exercise routine for his good health. He demonstrated a few of the thirty repetitions, moving his arms up and down to mimic using a five-pound weight to strengthen his upper body. Standing and stretching followed, complemented by walking—albeit with a walker because of his unsteadiness. "At the end of that, I feel very happy and good about myself and what I've accomplished."

"I'm really very regimented," he winked, and I realized that the order this gives his life—with daily doses of art, organ playing, and his physical "workouts"—helps to keep him young and vital. He agreed with my characterization, and just then the clocks chimed almost in unison. The hour allotted for the interview was up.

Henry was anxious to show me his artwork, so the wrap up took another half hour as he proudly took me through his home and showed me his newest art, a multi-layered creation made of paper, with elements of both a diorama and a collage appearing three-dimensional. Like his woodcarvings, they have depth but they are less demanding to work on. Perfect for this extraordinary ninety-six-year-old!

2 Julie: Botanical Watercolorist

Julie has come full circle. As a young girl and the oldest of seven children, she often accompanied her dad to his architecture office on Saturday mornings. She sat amidst large drafting tables with pencils and charcoal but never touched any of them. She didn't dare.

Her dad was well known in the Washington, DC, area where she grew up. He was also a talented amateur artist, she recalled, who returned to his first love, painting, when he retired. "He was a wonderful father but a little intimidating, and I never ever considered even drawing a line." She laughed as she glanced back affectionately into the distant past with the utmost respect for her father, much admired but too talented to emulate.

Now, at seventy-four and an accomplished botanical watercolorist with a current showing called *Beyond Words: The Symbolic Language of Plants* at the Delaware Art Museum, Julie can hardly believe her transformation. This is actually her second show: the first, in 2004, was a tribute to Lewis and Clark's transcontinental expedition from the Mississippi River to the west coast of Oregon. Commissioned by President Thomas Jefferson, its mission was to study the plant and animal life as well as the geography along the journey to learn what was economically viable. Julie's show was a tribute to the two-hundred-year anniversary of the expedition and featured botanical art created to replicate the newly discovered specimens that Lewis and Clark identified.

But, as you might suspect, a lot of water passed under the proverbial bridge before Julie came to her art. In fact, Julie believes that if her father hadn't been such an awesome role model to follow, or if he encouraged her in any way, she might have found the visual arts sooner. Until she was sixty-two, she confined her creativity to dabbling in crafts: sewing, embroidery, hanging wallpaper, handiwork of various sorts, but never fine arts. Her talent in school favored math, which was perfect for the shy and quiet young woman who became a computer programmer after completing an advanced degree in statistics.

Marrying her college sweetheart, supporting him through his Ph.D. program, and ultimately moving with him to Holland where his career took them defined the next phase of her life. This was a fairly typical scenario for young women of her era. Whatever her own unique talent might have been, it needed to take a back seat to her husband's career. Adulthood had its own set of challenges, as we well know, which Julie summarized in her matter-of-fact, logical way: "Make a home, raise two daughters, and live life as an active member of the community."

When her daughters were in college and after her divorce, she returned to Washington, DC, after almost twenty years to begin anew. Although her life until that point didn't include an art practice, she greatly benefitted from frequent visits to some of the finest museum collections in Holland and other European countries. She credited this exposure with an appreciation that informed her later work.

Back stateside and immersed in the activities of the church she attended as a child, Julie felt secure in the rhythm she created for herself by staying busy after work and finding her sea legs after an unsettling few years. Her now elderly father continued to paint and draw almost obsessively, but needed a fair amount of help in daily living. She was only too happy to oblige.

It gave her a chance to watch him in his studio and increasingly appreciate art, albeit still vicariously.

With barely enough time to catch her breath after retiring from her computer-programming job, Julie's father died. It was in cleaning out his huge basement studio that she got to see, examine, appreciate, and keep the tools of his trade. "I became curious about all of his things." I wondered whether this decision was driven by nostalgia to remember him or, possibly, to become more like him. "Now that I think of it, I was beginning to come out of a period when I was so busy taking care of him. I was curious, and I saw information about this class and I said, 'Okay, I'll do that.' The teacher had some drawings from her class pinned to the wall and I thought, 'That looks easy.'"

Her teacher's upbeat reaction made it more comfortable to take a leap of faith. As you might have guessed, this class was followed by many others in figure drawing, drawing with pastels, botanical drawing, and so on. "By the time I finished caring for my father and I was done with work, I wanted to take these art classes and I didn't care if I was the worst in the class. I've done lots of things I never dreamed I would do. I'm not afraid of failing. If I do, too bad. I'll try again. But I don't fail." We chatted about the benefits of the Vintage Years and the sense of freedom to try new things without worrying about judgments, along with more available time and increased ability to focus with fewer distractions.

"Art is a really big thing for me. The people I've met, the seventeen artists I work with—we've been together since 2004, since the Lewis and Clark Expedition exhibit. We're friends. We meet every Friday and paint together for three hours." These three hours mean so much more to her than simply creating art collectively. The people she's met are now part of her extended family, and through them the artistic community at large is a friendly, receptive place for this once shy girl.

I inquired about any additional time she devotes to art; she stated it was a daily routine. "I have a studio of my own in the basement. It's all my father's furniture." She lit up as she said this, as if she has incorporated her memory of her dad and his routines into her daily life. It occurred to me that one possible reason why her father was such an important influence on her life is that her mother died when she was nineteen.

I wanted to learn more about botanical drawing, and Julie was happy to oblige. "It started with a single flower in the middle of a white page, and now we're expanding the boundaries of botanical art." What began as rendering a true likeness of plants has, according to Julie, taken on more creativity, imagination, and artistry. "It's still realism," she explained as she described the center of a rose that might be greatly magnified but precise in its details.

I looked at the rendition of a blossoming crab apple tree branch in her current exhibit. This watercolor is extraordinarily accurate in its likeness, coloring, and size. The vivid golden pistils and stamens shine brightly in the center of each pale pink flower. A bee samples the nectar in one of the blooms. The surrounding leaves have variegated shades of green; the details of their scalloped edges and veins appear so real that they beckon my touch. Small, light green crab apples hang in the background, giving the blossoms their moment of splendor. With Julie's permission, I included a copy of one of her watercolors in the section featuring the work of those who contributed to the making of this book.

Julie mentioned a book written about an artist in the eighteenth century who created botanically precise images but expressed them in the form of paper cutouts set on pitch-black paper. What is especially fascinating from my viewpoint is that the artist, Mary Delaney, who was born in 1700, did not create this new art form, later called collage, until she was seventy-two and a newcomer to art. She worked at this process almost obsessively until her death at eighty-eight.

According to Mary Delaney's biographer, Molly Peacock, whose book reads like sumptuous poetry, "She painted large sheets of rag paper with watercolor, let them dry, then cut from them the hundreds of pieces she needed to reproduce—well, to re-evoke might be a better word—the flower she was portraying. There is no reproduced hue that matches the thrill of color in nature, yet Mrs. D. went after the original kick of natural color, and she did it like a painter.... But if you go to the British Museum's web site, zoom in on the image, then zoom in again and again, at last you will see the complicated overlapping layers of cut paper that this book shows in enlargements of details."[22]

The more my research takes me deeply into the lives of aging beginner artists, the more enthralling and awe-inspiring the process becomes. Digging still deeper to learn more about the con-connection between her current health and artistic undertaking, I asked Julie this question directly, as I did all the artists I interviewed. There is a growing body of evidence that playing a musical instrument later in life enhances posture and balance, and may reduce arthritic symptoms to say nothing of the beneficial stimulation to various parts of the brain. Many of the same

---

[22] *The Paper Garden*, pp. 7-8.

findings would apply to the visual arts, particularly for artists doing large-scale or three-dimensional work.

"I've always had good health, and I'm very energetic for my age," Julie responded. "That is largely genetic. But some personalities just keep going," she said, referring to her own personal style. While she doesn't credit her art with her enduring health, she acknowledged that some of her artist friends who have less robust health continue to express their artistry, which enhances their lives and makes life worth living notwithstanding the limitations.

As we began to wind down, Julie offered some advice for others just getting started. "You just keep doing things and eventually you get into something. I had already decided that I wasn't going to sit around and wait for something to happen." She suggested that the starting point is not so important, because from that first step evolves interest and even passion that carries energy and momentum, making the process sublime even without an eventual goal. But she emphasized the need for the best instruction that one can afford. For Julie, that meant a rather pricey private art school. The cost was a stretch for her—she laughed as she said, "Believe me, if you have to pay $800, you're not going to miss class, and you get there on time!" According to Julie, a good teacher "helps you be successful step-by-step, and it helps a lot if you have people in the class who are really serious about it." She found that some of the community programs were not as well organized and less serious in their approach.

Though her second exhibit is barely underway, Julie is looking forward to her next step—an oil painting class and wherever that takes her.

3 Marty: Bronze Sculptor

A scrappy, sharp-witted kid, Marty grew up on Coney Island in Brooklyn, New York. His family was in the pinball machine business. His father and uncle distributed and serviced these machines all over the city and later owned a penny arcade in Coney Island, which anyone over sixty can picture. He remembered the long work hours and personally vowed to avoid becoming a shopkeeper. That was many years ago.

Marty's web site previewed his talent and zest for life. I looked at it before our meeting; it testified to his science-philosopher-artist nature. I felt prepared to meet this extraordinary man, but our meeting happened in a rather peculiar way. With computer-generated map and directions in hand, I wound my way up a scenic hill toward his home, confident in my ability to follow directions only to become lost—a rather embarrassing situation.

Since I was going to be late, I called. Marty answered in the take-charge way that I soon discovered was a key to understanding him. I provided the street coordinates that defined my location; he asked me to stay put, as I was only a few blocks away. He said to expect his gray SUV to appear in about two minutes, and he was soon there. As I later quipped, this was the first time I ever followed a strange man home!

Home was a California ranch-style abode buried in the trees so that its façade was hard to take in with a single glance. It seemed like the perfect environment for a sculptor. Sitting by the front door was a once-upon-a-time olive tree, now sculpted into the likeness of a family of three people—or as a sculptor might say, released from the tree.

At eighty-four, Marty has the appearance and energy of a much younger man. His wiry build benefits from going to the gym two days a week. His fitness routine may be necessary to maintain his ability to wrestle with three-foot-high chunks of alabaster. On the other hand, regular workouts are part of the well-thought-out weekly plan for the life of this retired executive. A weekly sculpture class has been another regular event on his calendar for years. In fact, when asked how he started and maintains his art practice, Marty summed up how he tackles most things. "Just do it. Don't just talk about it or wish you would do it. If you don't join a class, you won't do it." His words came out forcefully and convincingly. He has no patience for people who yearn but don't act.

Marty's art did not get started in a just-do-it way at all. We sat at his kitchen table as he poured steaming coffee in my cup and urged me to have another cookie. His wife, Lee, joined us at the table, and he asked her to tell what turned out to be a prophetic tale. Lee explained that shortly after they were married, in their early twenties, she decided to introduce him to some culture in the form of museums, concerts, ballets, and other civilizing influences. Marty cued her to recall their first trip to an art museum.

I could see she was trying to remember back, not sure which anecdote he wanted her to tell. Then, she brightened up when her memory registered, and she began to speak. "We would walk in, and he would see a sculpture by, I don't know, some famous artist, and he would say, 'I can do that.' And I would say, 'Are you kidding?' And then he'd see another sculpture and say, 'I can do that.' And finally, I stopped and said, 'Look, this is not like taking some clay and making stuff for the kids, these are great sculptures.' He replied, 'Why can't I do that?'" Lee laughed as she recalled the comical conversation: "Marty just repeated, 'So what's the big deal? I can do that.'" When I asked if he actually did do it after all, the answer was an emphatic no!

I marveled at his sureness regarding something he knew nothing about. Marty chimed in, laughing as he recalled a conversation from roughly sixty years ago. "I just knew if I wanted to, I could do it." Maybe catching himself sounding arrogant, he quickly added that he didn't think he could do any other art form, like painting or ceramics; he could just do sculpture. His long-ago proclamations to his wife were soon forgotten, and he never thought about sculpting again until 1982. Life happened: children were born and grew up; Marty's career developed; and time went on.

As he told his story, Marty's eyes appeared to get heavy and his voice softened. His breathing seemed to slow and his ready-for-action body sagged a bit as he explained how his art evolved slowly out of profound sadness and grief following his eighteen-year-old son's suicide in 1981. "That destroyed everything," Marty said. Details didn't follow; it seemed inappropriate to inquire. He moved on quickly to the saving grace provided by his career as Research Director of Pharmacology in a pharmaceutical company from 1960–1985. Immersion in his work provided some distraction and time away from the devastation and suffering that he and his family experienced.

His voice and demeanor began to pick up as he talked about 1983. "It was an incredible, unbelievable accident. I picked up a newspaper that I never read and haven't since. I was looking down at ads, and there was an ad for a sculpture class. I never read that newspaper, never looked at those ads, but for some reason my eye caught that ad. I was trying to come back to the world. And I looked at it and said, 'I always wanted to. Maybe.' I called the guy up, a nice Italian guy from Bayonne, New Jersey, and said, 'Angelo, I never took an art class in my life. I don't know what this is all about, but I want to do it.' He was so encouraging over the phone that I went home and said, 'I never did this before, but I am going to take this week off to take these classes down in Santa Cruz.' There were ten people in the class: three professional artists, three art teachers, and three others who had some experience. I was the only man. During that week, I began to perceive that my work was easily in the top third of the class, and some students were professionals!"

With a twinkle in his eye and nostalgia in his voice, Marty recalled wondering on the first day of class, "What the hell am I doing here? The assistant laid out some materials, and then I look over, and she's standing stark naked on the table. Hey, what goes on here?" he laughed. "Lunchtime was a big event; Angelo was big on lunch, and lunch lasted a European two hours. I found myself in an outdoor café in Santa Cruz, having lunch and a glass of wine with this girl who was stark naked a few minutes ago, and now she's sitting right next to me talking, laughing, and telling stories. And, I wasn't looking at my watch to see what time we had to get back." Marty quipped again, "What the hell was this?" "Like an alternative reality," I offered. He nodded, as if from a distance, as if he was still at lunch in Santa Cruz. "What an experience," he concluded.

We came back to the present moment, a bit jolting after the trip down memory lane. I suggested that a one-week course, even if a peak experience, is hard to build on. After Santa Cruz, Marty had difficulty finding classes close to home and tried a ceramics class, which he attacked in his intense, compulsive, and driven way. "But it wasn't sculpture."

In Marty's precise and detailed style, he laid out the chronology of art classes that followed intermittently. "Every once in a while, I would say, 'I'm leaving. Goodbye. I'm going to take a one week class.' Those were very good experiences." He would fly to Colorado or Arizona for a week and meet people from everywhere, which he reveled in as the engaging, outgoing, sociable person that he is. When I inquired how he kept his interest alive between classes, he acknowledged that he could not. When I came back, that was the end of it." I pointed out that he had two identities: the full-time corporate guy and the part-time artist, straddling the two worlds for a while.

It was not until 1990, when he was sixty-three and retired from full-time work, that he became serious about his art and he found a local weekly class that became his Wednesday morning ritual, which he continues to this day. It has morphed into an open studio—the same place and materials but without instruction. While the place is important, he asserted, "These people became very close friends. This core group has been a very important part of my life." He repeats this statement to emphasize just how important this community continues to be in his life.

Focusing next on the experience and emotion of creating art, Marty said, "You can be working for three hours and disappear and get totally lost in what you're doing." I suspect that his absorption into sculpting helped him survive and thrive in the years following his son's death. These days, getting lost in his art leads to creative breakthroughs, like when he moved from sculpting clay to sculpting stone. "I'm moving now from what I would call the additive, where you add clay to build a shape, to the subtractive, where you take away from stone and wood." I suggested that the novelty in his new approach may stimulate his brain, which is one of my hypotheses about how the arts benefit the aging brain. "Absolutely," he chimes in with emphasis, "Some of my classmates are experiencing the same thing—the feeling that we've got to move on and do something different." Marty feels that "the subtractive method of sculpting wood and stone is more intellectually challenging," confirming that problem solving also stimulates the brain to function optimally.

Regarding motivation and staying power, Marty reminded me that "over the years, people have said to me, 'Oh, I always wanted to do this painting' or, 'I have a set of paints in my closet,' and I tell people, 'If you don't join a class, you are not going to do it.'" He repeats this sentence twice for emphasis and is adamant that I must include "Marty's mantra" in my book. He goes on: "I don't care how self-motivated you are, I certainly qualify as a very highly-motivated type of person. I'm a classic A-type, which I laugh about. No matter how self-motivated I am, if I don't put it on the calendar, I'll find a million excuses to not do it."

We talked about accountability and regularity, and ways to keep the art going forward. Marty sees his class as similar to going to the gym: "You need to do it; like sit-ups; like piano scales; or like working at the barre if you do ballet. Many times I say to myself, 'I don't know what the hell I'd be doing if I didn't take up sculpture.' I could have gotten involved in a volunteer organization." He suddenly trails off, then leaps up, moves to a cabinet flanking his studio, hops up so that he is sitting on it, and eagerly shows me the books about sculpture that he has accumulated over the years. "Look at all of the wonderful artists' lives I've learned about. Look at all the history of art I've learned about, all part of life that was nonexistent for me as a child." A whole new world had opened up to Marty, who came from a pragmatic, working-class family who regarded the arts as more or less irrelevant.

He went on to describe the excitement he experienced learning the bronze process. "Here's the bronze process that's four thousand years old, and learning every facet of the bronze process became fascinating. I found a boutique foundry where I could put on the boots and the mask and become part of the process. Now I'm welding! Sculpture absolutely enriched my life."

I suggested to him that some of the readers of this book won't be like him: energized and excited just waking up in the morning. Others might not be able to identify with his experience. Is there hope for them? He reiterated his mantra: "Join that class. You wake up in the morning, and you know the class is starting at nine-thirty in the morning, so you get out of bed."

Although he rejected my idea of legacy as a motivation for his art, Marty will be remembered by members of the Jewish temple he belongs to for the bronzed continuous-loop torah that he created and donated, and that became the central focus of a meditation garden built around it. He will be remembered.

I could see that Marty had the energy to continue our conversation endlessly, but we moved instead to a tour of his home and his studio, where most of his art is displayed. He has no real interest in selling his art pieces, although several won juried events. One piece was selected for a memorial ceremony commemorating the first anniversary of the 2001 World Trade Center disaster. He is nonchalant but orderly in his review, moving methodically from his first works—some clay nymphs now clustered around an indoor koi pond—to his latest work: a pinkish alabaster piece, about three feet high, that seems lit from the inside. But that is the beauty of Marty's art.

4 Gene: Landscape Painter

"I grew up in New York City, Greenwich Village in fact, which had some impact on me. An older cousin of mine lived in Brooklyn and used to paint in the basement of his home. I was immediately taken by my cousin's painting and the smell of the paint. I hadn't known what an impact that made until the closing of the first chapter of my life and I could look forward to painting. How potent that experience was! I went through a career with that percolating in me, and it bubbled up when I started to think about retirement and could see a way to do it. I began to have some anger about the possibility of dying too soon—running out of time. I expected to have forever after I retired so that I could paint. So far, I'm relieved." These are Gene's words in the first five minutes of our interview as we crossed the threshold to the living room where his cousin's larger-than-life paintings hang on the walls.

Transplanted to California, he retains his New York accent, which intensified my own when we spoke. At eighty, his speech is soft but precise as he describes his health; he ranked it between good and excellent on the one-page questionnaire I asked him to complete. He approached the questionnaire in a serious way, thinking about his answers before he wrote them. I realized that this might be an artifact of his long career as a psychologist writing psychological reports for many years—understanding the impact of words on the reader. But I digress.

Regarding his birthplace, Greenwich Village is a very artistic community. The 1950s were a particularly interesting time there—beatnik artists, poets, and musicians everywhere you looked. Living there, however, didn't help Gene's artistic development. "The little art I did in school," said Gene, "was considerably unimaginative, and I was inhibited, so that dissuaded me from doing art."

When he was ten, his mother took Gene, along with a horse he had modeled out of clay, to see a neighbor artist for some feedback about his ability. The artist was polite but not encouraging, a common-enough scenario—few mentors existed for those not recognized as gifted. We know that childhood is often not the time for artistry to flourish. But as he grew older, he became interested in doodling, and while he thought he was reasonably good and maybe had some talent, he never developed art as a hobby until his Vintage Years. For fifty-four years, Gene carried that potent olfactory memory of the paint smell in his cousin's Brooklyn studio. He didn't actually begin to paint until he retired as the chief psychologist at the VA Palo Alto Healthcare System.

Being a psychologist myself, I was well aware that retirement is always optional. Psychology is a profession in which people frequently work very late into life. We both laughed when I suggested that so long as we could hear and sit on a chair, we could continue working. Gene volunteered that before his mid sixties, he felt restless and could no longer feel any kicks from what he was doing. He was ready for a change and not anxious or worried about what would come next. "I knew that I was going to retire at some point, and I knew that when I did, I would start to paint. I tend to throw myself into things fully." His one concern was how that would affect his relationship with his wife, who might have been seeking a playmate rather than an artist husband who would disappear into his studio for hours or days.

Gene and his wife took a vacation to mark his retirement at sixty-four; he knew in advance when the trip would be and hence how to time his retirement. Precise in his planning, as is his nature, he explained, "As soon as we got back, I enrolled in classes." His preparation was apparently seamless. I questioned how he knew how to get started, where to find classes, and such. Gene relished doing his homework in advance and knew about the local art league and community center. Before he retired he stopped in to look around. "Most of my training was done there and on an occasional foray elsewhere for a workshop."

I could imagine his experience as a newbie painter. This was a man accustomed to being at the top of his profession and considered an expert with superior accomplishments. "What was it like for you to start all over?" I queried. He replied, "It was frustrating for me. I was used to performing well. I was a decent basketball player when I was a kid, and I expected myself to be better at art than it turns out I was." I wondered out loud whether that shook his resolve to paint. He laughed and said, "There was no question in my mind. If I stunk, then I'd enjoy stinking!" He hesitated, looking serious and deep in thought about his next words before he went on: "I consider myself a tolerable amateur."

I suggested that this is a stage of life in which achievement takes a back seat to pleasure and asked what he gets out of his art. "I get satisfaction from a painting that I've done that meets my standards, where I can say, 'Okay, it's finished.'" I tried to get to the feeling that underpins his observation that while he points to the pleasure of a job well done, he also recognizes that the process is hard work. "I try to solve painting problems that constantly remind me how minimally trained and skilled I am, how little I know." I reminded him that problem solving in art is one of those things that keeps the neurons firing. It's a brain workout. He agrees that challenging himself with the increasing complexity of his projects is healthy. In the end, he is self-satisfied and happy.

"I evolved to the open studio where you go to draw or paint live models. I wanted to be good at figures, but it turned out I wasn't. So I focused on painting landscapes, and when I could carry most of my gear outdoors to do *pleinairy*[23], I did. But as time went by, I was too tired to paint after schlepping all of my stuff. As long as I had enough exposure to landscape possibilities, I was not bereft."

Gene continued to accommodate his changing limitations as he grew older, now painting landscapes from sketches and from photos that he takes while traveling, which is another lifelong interest finally being fulfilled. But he was quick to add that he returned to face and figure drawing and is now taking another class. "I'm doing something new; I want to conquer an old failure," meaning his difficulty in painting the human body when he first started painting fifteen years ago. I reiterated my mantra that doing something new keeps the brain alert and sharp. It's a tonic for the brain, just like problem solving, and it creates what neuroscience researchers call cognitive reserve.

We discussed the inevitable age-related changes that are natural and normal. Slower response time, increased difficulty in retrieving the right word, and diminished physical strength are

---

[23] Pleinairy comes from the French expression *en plein air*, which can be translated as "in the open air" and refers to the practice of painting outdoors.

typical but manageable. Because I see fine-tuning the body and mind as critical to our development as Vintage-stage artists, I've provided some strategies about ways to adapt and compensate. Look for them under the subheading, "Synergy: Wisdom, Exercise, and the Brain" in Chapter 8.

There is ample evidence that you can do your art even when other faculties fail, even if you are limited in expressing yourself verbally. These limitations do not need to impede writing, painting, or playing a musical instrument. "It's continually available," Gene comments about his art, "with very little pressure from your body to have to give it up." Clearly, he's in it for the long haul, adapting his art to his changing needs and interests.

Other than the occasional trip, need for a change of scene, or shopping foray, Gene paints daily. His guest-room-turned-office is also his studio, where he painstakingly works through a problem in executing his painting or gets lost in it completely. When it's going well, he emerges refreshed and happy.

Sometimes, Gene's wife, Ziva, gives him critical feedback on a sketch or painting—a reality check, he says—that brings him down to earth. But, his art brings newness to their relationship and informs their lifestyle as well. They spend more time together in venues that are creative and artistic, and her support of his artwork is invaluable. So much for the earlier worries about how his painting in retirement would affect their relationship!

When we said our goodbyes, I asked for a few final words of wisdom to help guide prospective retirees who may not be too sure about their futures. "If you can't imagine what you want to do when you retire, and you enjoy what you are doing, I'd say, find a way to keep doing it." Remembering his perspective and his experience, this advice makes sense. It does, however, differ from the advice of others who simply dived into the deep end of an unfamiliar pool and learned something new about themselves in the process.

5 Betsy: Ceramicist

It was a bright summer afternoon in the hills of northern California when we met at Betsy's modest California ranch-style house. The winding road led to a heavily populated neighborhood with other small ranch-style homes, probably built in the 50s. This was a community of working people and their families.

Having heard about my project from a mutual acquaintance, Betsy must have given this interview a lot of thought, because she consulted with her sister at length about whether to volunteer for my study. Her sister's enthusiastic response provided the impetus: "You helped me see that I could retire without a plan. I think you should share your experience to inspire others to do the same." And so she did.

Now sixty-six, Betsy is tall and slender. With a quiet voice, she speaks in a determined way. She ushered me into her open-plan living room, dim in contrast to the afternoon sun, and gestured that I take a chair across from her. The sofa on which she sat was covered in light-colored towels, seeming odd until her miniature poodle came flying around the corner to inspect the situation and took his place beside her. She smiled as she explained the origin of Madison's name and previewed how he would vie for attention during the ensuing hour. He's a dog who is used to getting what he wants, and Betsy did a good job picking up on his cues.

Finally, getting down to business, Betsy started with the end of her career. She took a permanent disability leave at fifty-five after a lengthy career as a research physicist. It was a sudden change that left her a bit shell-shocked. This was the first time in her life that she didn't know her next step. Being thrown into retirement by illness gave her no time to prepare, plan, or execute—the very opposite of how scientists work. Sadness crossed her face like a shadow as she told about this uncomfortable time in her life. As a single woman, whose work was at the center of her daily life, the void swallowed her identity.

A few emotionally and physically taxing years passed. As Betsy began to recover some strength, she turned to photography, which had once been an on-again-off-again hobby. Going through the motions helped her pass time, and trying the local photo club did give her some of the contact with people that she craved. But, she felt no passion or cohesiveness around which to build a new life. Photography lacked the spark to ignite her future.

Then came the succulent society phase, when she thought that creating a California-style water-wise garden would be a good thing. "My neighbor turned me on to this. I wanted to get out and meet people. So I went to the succulent society meeting twice, and it just wasn't my cup of tea. I did learn something from one of the speakers—how to keep the deer from eating your garden. But at the end of each meeting there was a competition. People brought in a plant that they wanted to show off, and competition is not my thing."

The one-upmanship permeating the group made her feel uncomfortable and unwelcome. This turned out to be another dead end. The knitting guild was the next venue in her search for satisfaction, maybe even passion, and community. Both of her sisters knitted, so she thought this might be a good choice for her. She threw herself into meetings, workshops, and projects, and met some people with whom she continues to socialize, but like her earlier activities, this was not a perfect choice. As she describes it, the process was "a bit too meticulous, too precise."

More time passed as Betsy continued to look around for an interest that combined the right mix of challenge and interest. She was sixty-two. Nearly seven years had passed since disability retirement was forced on her, and at this point she felt like she was "going downhill."

Her discovery of ceramics was entirely accidental and almost didn't happen at all. "So, when I was thinking, 'this is going downhill,' I got a catalogue in the mail from the city recreation center. Usually, they don't send it here." She explained it was probably delivered by mistake. Just as she was about to toss it into the recycling bin, she glanced at it and for some reason looked at the list of the upcoming classes. She saw one that was interesting, a beginning ceramics class, but since she wasn't a resident of the town, she would have lowest priority at registration. For some inexplicable reason, she was compelled to be first at the registration site after locals had registered. And sure enough, she got in! That was the beginning of her love affair with ceramics. "I thought it might be fun, and I've been doing it ever since." She looked at me and smiled, her face flushing with pleasure. "Yeah, it was a find!"

How did she know to pursue this particular art form about which she knew absolutely nothing? "It's like in science when they talk about the prepared mind," she replied. "These people who made the big discoveries—their minds were ready with all the information, and when the last thing kicked into place, it was POW!" She gestured with her hand, like a rocket taking off, as she explained that in science a breakthrough is not really accidental.

I loved the concept of the prepared mind, which explains so much of what I observed when those I interviewed described finally selecting an art to pursue with passion. "I was serious; I really wanted this to happen. Part of it was the ceramics and part was the very nice people I met there." I suggested that she was looking for something with her prepared mind and ceramics had that magical quality of a hand fitting perfectly into a glove.

Looking back and reminiscing, Betsy tried to paint a cohesive picture of her life and also explain why ceramics was the perfect fit for her. She grew up in a family that valued science and education; her father was a physician and her mother a nurse. It was natural for her to follow on this path. Her science potential was evident early, despite the fact that she had trouble reading—much later she diagnosed herself as dyslexic. In her sixties, she finally understood why ceramics, a three-dimensional art, was a good fit for a dyslexic mind.

When asked about her interest in any of the fine arts as a child or adolescent, she laughed and recalled that at the end of fourth grade, she went to camp and made a hat out of paper. At the time, she didn't make the connection between the hat and her affinity for a three-dimensional art form, so that ended her artistic exploration until the photography phase began in her fifties. It's now evident that she couldn't capture on paper what she saw in the camera lens, which was frustrating for her. Now she understands—photography is a two-dimensional art.

That first ceramics class introduced her to clay and building objects from all angles. The feel of the cool clay, the ability to mold it, shape it, play with it, and understand its three-dimensional form was all part of its attraction. The people she encountered felt like kindred spirits. "They made me feel welcome." Betsy finally felt at home.

Courses led to workshops and time spent in an open studio where she could practice what she learned for hours and further refine her tastes and techniques. Curiosity, and the search for more complexity along with her budding skill, led her to add the local community college as an art venue. This turned out to be the perfect place to continue developing her skill and to feed her intellectually curious mind.

"Because of my scientific background, when there was a problem with one of the glazes, I looked into why that might be. It was a question, and it was interesting, and to make a long story short, if I could add a few more percent of this certain chemical that might solve it, and so I did that, and sure enough it fixed it."

Not only did Betsy experience a lot of satisfaction, she also came to be known as the glaze guru. "I'm always being asked to weigh out glazes because I'm accurate." Now when things are wrong with the glazes, Betsy is called upon to fix it, which requires research that's right up her alley. "What I liked about science and research was figuring things out and taking different bits of information and synthesizing it into something." I reflected that this sounded like problem solving, which my research has shown is one of the things that keeps the brain young. Dealing with increasing complexity and novel situations leads to greater production of neurons and links between neurons.

Betsy explained that timing is everything in art, as it is in science. "One of the things I learned is that you've got to do it when the clay is ready to do it, which means you've got to be there, not once a week or twice a week. Do a little bit and let it rest, and come back the next day and do a little more. So I set up a place in my kitchen where I can work on pieces. I can do it whenever I want to, so the clay and I are in sync." Later, as she showed me her workplace and finished art, I realized that not only does she enjoy the process of doing the art, but she gets a kick out of looking at the finished pieces that decorate her home. She laughed at my conceptualization and readily agreed with my summing up.

An interesting by-product of her ceramics involvement is that it benefits her health and stamina. Was it the physical nature of wrestling with clay? Was it getting used to the climb up a steep hill from the parking lot to the college? Was it the love for what she was doing that led unexpectedly to the physical conditioning that improved her health? The cause-and-effect relationship is hard to untangle and probably not necessary, but the outcome is better health and a more positive outlook at this point in time. What began as "a way to get me out of the house" has become a way of life.

As she signs my release form and I gather my paraphernalia to leave, Betsy sums things up. "I love it! I'm passionate about ceramics and very happy with my life." I threw just one more question her way about how others might get started. She quickly noted, "Number one, don't prejudge any of the possibilities until you try them. It may disappoint you or it may vastly exceed your expectations. Number two, talk to people. You never know who's going to have the idea that is the thing."

6 Harold: Stained Glass Artist

This New York City native looked so young that when he told me he was eighty-six years old, I did a double take. He's not the kind of man to get plastic surgery, so I'd like to think that wrestling with big pieces of glass, making just the right cuts, fitting the pieces together, and edging them with copper foil is the type of workout that keeps you looking your best. Harold is a stained glass artist.

He still seemed surprised as he told me his story. We sat in his modern-style living room in the home he shares with his wife of many years. Like most of the people I interviewed, Harold had no history in the arts, no training other than what kids learn in big-city public schools. We quickly glossed over his growing-up years, typical of boys in that time and place but not especially relevant to his current artistry. Like almost all the men I interviewed, his adult life centered on home, family, children, and work—in his case, sales in the gourmet food business. He joked as we looked for any possible link between his line of work and his current artistic life. We found none. During the middle of his adult life, he spent any spare time building and fixing things at home. Working with his hands was important then and continues to be now.

During their forties, Harold and his wife enjoyed spending weekends going to antique fairs, sometimes looking, sometimes buying for their personal use. On one such occasion, they bought four stained glass windows salvaged from a demolished church in Connecticut. "I sold two that were not in perfect shape but cleaned up the frames for the other two and installed them in my dining room. The stained glass was so striking that when we later sold our home to move to this place (in New Jersey), the sale was contingent on the stained glass remaining behind!" It seemed prophetic that his love for the stained glass windows materialized into a hobby, though not until much later.

At sixty-five, Harold and his wife moved to their retirement home. "I was busy doing things, repairing things, hanging wallpaper, hanging fixtures. Once that was finished, I ended up doing nothing. I was always handy but never did any stained glass. I never did art. I really can't draw," he said with great emphasis and some wistfulness in his voice. "I had to have something to do and saw that there were art courses in the local high school at night, so I signed up for a stained glass course. When I took the course, I felt that I found something that I could do.

"So I stayed with it and started making little things, and as I made them, I started giving them away to friends, and they liked them very much. I went on to bigger things, like making stained glass windows for my garage door. I tried some innovative techniques that no one else was doing, and it came out beautifully." His expression had changed. Harold was energized by his story. As he reflected on the past twenty years, his face beamed and his words came faster, as if he might run out of time before finishing.

I asked Harold what he got out of doing his art, and he responded as if the words were on the tip of his tongue, "Great satisfaction and not only that, compliments. To me, when I give something to someone and they like it, it's worth all the work I put into it. I love the compliments." What started out as personally satisfying is now also highly reinforced by others' appreciation.

As time went by, the size and scope of his projects grew from small to large windows and then doors. A studio was added to his house, a sunroom resembling the ones you see in nurseries where fragile, hothouse plants grow. Even when it's twenty degrees outside, Harold works comfortably in his studio. In the summer, when hot houses are even hotter, Harold gets up before the sun to begin his glasswork.

As his reputation spread, he was asked to make stained glass windows for the nearby synagogue. "Four of them were to go on a light box; it was a large and complex project." He wound up having to create the difficult design, this artist who at one time could not draw!

Suddenly, Harold launched into great detail about cutting, edging, and assembling that project. He spoke like the teacher he had become, perhaps so caught up in reliving the experience or thinking about me as if I were his student that the lecture went way over my head. He felt it was an honor to be asked by the rabbi, so he did the work gratis, charging only for materials.

The accolades that came his way still sustain him. He knows he likes the positive attention and understands how it motivates his work. Like virtually all of the extroverts I interviewed, the adulation from an appreciative audience energizes and incentivizes. Introverts are mostly content with their own experience and self-acknowledgement and don't require an external audience.

Because the synagogue window project was such a success, ten additional windows were requested. "Which came out gorgeous," he said without modesty, "and now there are fifteen stained glass windows, in total, around this small temple." I commented that it must have looked like the Sistine Chapel. He responded, "I never thought about myself as doing something like this. I'm a very simple person."

If Harold were ever a simple person, it must have been a long time ago. During the past twenty years, he has demonstrated his ability to learn very complex artistic processes and to execute them so finely that his work decorates homes and places of worship for miles around. Most of all, he enjoys his time and is proud of the legacy he's leaving for others to enjoy. "I know I'm aging because my body tells me that I am, but I refuse to slow down, because the art—I can do it. I can't walk so fast, I can't run, and I can't pick up as much as I used to. But as long as I can do this, I'm very happy."

As we finished the tour of his sunroom workshop, he directed my attention to a small mirror encased in stained glass right in front of me. He asked if I liked it. The long handle had beautifully carved and intricate flowers seemingly twined on a vine. It was lovely and reminded me of the kind you associate with Sleeping Beauty or Snow White, sitting at their dressing tables brushing their hair. Harold picked up the mirror and handed it to me. As I turned it over and admired both sides he said, "It's yours!" Before I had a chance to protest, Harold found a sturdy box and some bubble wrap to insure its safe passage back to California. It now adorns my dresser, and I smile warmly when I think of Harold at work in his sunroom, surrounded by intensely bright and colorful glass pieces waiting to be joined.

7 Judy: Watercolorist

Judy describes herself as a chronically busy person, so it was no surprise that pinpointing a meeting time proved challenging. The first-ever art studio showing of her watercolor paintings preempted our initial attempt. Our next date was affected by a call from the hospital where she does per diem work as a social worker as needed, and she was needed. But finally we found a date, and I drove to her home in Portola Valley, nestled in the wilderness and rimmed by the coastal mountain range in northern California.

Because the dry months of California's Mediterranean climate cause the grass to yellow, I was struck by the vast expanse of bright gold as I drove deep into the valley. Though the first rain of the season was taking place that very day, the yellowed meadows would not benefit this year. Next spring it will be very green again.

Judy's modern, wood-sided house, tucked into the scenery and surrounded by California native trees like the coastal oak, almost looked like it grew out of the surrounding vegetation. Even without an artist's eye, this scene looked like a fine painting, notwithstanding the rain. It was ironic that the landscape, softened by the early fall rain, resembled a watercolor, the very genre that I was going to learn more about shortly.

Judy was born and raised in Boston. Every summer, from the time she was a young child, her family went to their cottage-by-the-sea in Rockport, Massachusetts, a small artist's colony, originally a lobster-fishing town. "During all of those years, I never had the urge to paint," she recalled. At sixty-six, she continues to return year after year to Rockport in the summer, nowadays spending time with her three siblings at this much-loved, peaceful, and calming place filled with family memories from the past.

On a typical visit nine years ago, she was doing what she has done on numerous occasions—stopping at art galleries. Looking at paintings always has and still does give her tremendous pleasure. But this time, she wondered to herself what it would be like to paint. It was just a passing thought, as Judy had never thought about painting before and up until that point had no history of training or experience other than looking and appreciating. As we know, all children are exposed to art and various art projects early in life through school, but most don't make it a career or even a serious hobby. Judy was no exception.

She was fifty-seven when her curiosity was activated in that art gallery in Rockport. She thought, "Maybe I'll take one of the drop-in classes," referring to the offerings of local artists who supplement their incomes by teaching. "So I went to a local toy store and bought one of these kid's watercolor sets and a pad. I wanted to try watercolor because it wasn't messy. It's not like oils, where you have to have turpentine—it smells—and you have to have a real studio and do it outside. I thought, 'I don't want to deal with that.'" She laughed as she related her very pragmatic approach to picking an art medium. "Besides," she added, "I just love watercolors." "Why?" I asked, which is not an easy question to answer. "It's flowing," she replied. "I like the transparency and the way the colors mix in a very subtle way. Once I started doing it, I realized that there is something magical and very soothing about water colors."

We went on to talk about the feel of the art, which she described as almost meditative, although Judy has never formally learned to meditate, so she dismissed that idea. I disagreed, and suggested that this IS her form of meditation, a kind of moving meditation. She listened and then nodded in agreement, as if she finally had a name for the spiritual state she finds herself in while painting.

She recalled her first class. "I was very, very absorbed in what I was doing, and the time went by just like that." She snapped her fingers and emphasized her surprise at the end of the class. She was hooked! The rest is history. After the first class in Rockport, she continued back in California at the community art center and city adult education program. Like virtually all of my interviewees, she emphasized the importance of continuing to take classes. Nine years later, she is still taking classes and working on her own pieces the rest of the time.

Judy had an uncanny way of anticipating and answering my questions before I even asked them. In writing this book, I am seeking ways to understand how the aging brain facilitates the development of artistic expression later in life, and conversely how artistic expression stimulates the aging brain. Judy seemed to understand intuitively how this worked for her, and she went on to explain it.

When she entered her fifties, coinciding with menopause, she began to feel more independent of the influences that had shaped her life from the outside. Her mother and maternal grandmother were strong, independent, and very ambitious women. Way ahead of their times, her mother was a newspaper reporter and her grandmother was the first woman delegate to the World Health Organization. "That female script in my family was very powerful." But it struck her that "I don't have to be ambitious. When I turned fifty, I said. 'Damn it. This is not me.

This is my mother talking. I can do things for their own sake,' and I began to feel more comfortable psychologically and physically. I actually had more energy. It really just hit me, and my life has been better since then."

We wondered if her shifting attitude about doing things that pleased her, rather than achieving in order to prove herself to the outside world, prepared her to embrace the artist's life still to come. I suggested that when she turned fifty, she freed herself from the shackles that bound her until then, and she nodded enthusiastically. "I'm not very judgmental about what I do. It's really the process that grabs me, and I love it. I was pretty bad, but I just didn't care." At this time in her life, she's accepting of her creations; this acceptance allowed her to pursue art in the first place.

Judy's awareness about her internal changes is consistent with other mid-life people who sense a shift in their perception of what's important. Some of this is hormonal, in her case a decrease in estrogen, which I discussed in Chapter 3. Some of the shift occurs because of the brain's structural and chemical changes related to a consolidation of a lifetime of learning that is better known as wisdom. More about wisdom can be found in Chapter 8.

Training and experience as a psychiatric social worker may have been the impetus for Judy to talk candidly and directly about her own psychological tendencies to worry and over-think situations that are bothersome. For her, one of the wonders of painting is that her head is now filled with projects and problems to be solved about current or future watercolor ventures. For example, Judy replayed a typical situation we've all encountered—being stopped in a traffic jam on the freeway. In the past, she would have worried about her kids or grandkids, often about issues that were not rational or under her control.

When you have a tendency to worry, it's like that. The fearful what-ifs push to the surface of consciousness and grow like plants in early spring—they shoot up and become very large with minimal work. Judy thinks painting is the solution. Nowadays, when she is lost in thought, daydreaming, or stuck in traffic with an idling car, her mind is full. She might be looking out the car window at a scene she'd love to capture on canvas, or the shadows cast by the angle of the sun, or the book she created with watercolors illustrating a handwritten story she's working on for her grandson—or any number of pleasant thoughts. Even when she goes into her problem-solving mode, she's most likely focused on ways to overcome a technical artistic problem, like the church tower in her most recent painting that appears to be leaning slightly.

Judy didn't take up art to manage her busy, worrisome mind; her initial curiosity, reinforced by interest and later by passion, led her to it. But, one huge benefit was that it re-oriented the content of her thinking away from fearful what-ifs and toward the wonders of art. Perhaps because of this, she says she is a much happier person.

To prove how fully absorbed she becomes while painting, she told the following story. About two years ago, she was on the way to her evening painting class when she had a fall and landed right on her kneecap. She vacillated about whether to go home and rest it or go to class where she sat on a high stool with her legs dangling. She opted for class although her knee had begun to throb.

She described herself being so focused during class, so totally immersed in the art, that she was oblivious to what was going on around her, even apparently inside of her. When it was time to leave and as she packed up, she "felt the worse pain that I've felt in my entire life, and I looked down. My knee was swollen up like a cantaloupe, and that's not an exaggeration. Somehow, I managed to get home, but was literally screaming on the way to the emergency room when my husband took me there. But the entire time I was painting, I had felt nothing!" She emphasized *nothing* in amazement. "I was completely anesthetized!"

We marveled at the experience of being so fully involved that even pain is muted. While an extreme example, Judy feels that in general, her art takes her away from all cares and concerns. When she emerges from a painting session, she feels calm, peaceful, and content. There's one additional benefit according to her.

Judy's memory for and ability to retrieve words became more difficult following menopause. Like many post-menopausal women and some older men, remembering the names of people, places, and things can become a challenge. But, this challenge doesn't affect her watercolor painting at all. Artistic expression doesn't depend on this verbal skill. Whether painting, writing, or playing a musical instrument, an art form once learned is for life!

8 Dan: Full-Time Art Student

Dan will finish his four-year art school degree in a couple of months. His bachelor's degree in Fine Arts doesn't provide any direction after graduation. He prefers sculpting and thinks he'll take a bronze-casting class next fall. He's not concerned with how to make a living or market his art to the public. He's laid-back about his future and takes one day at a time.

He may sound to you like the typical twenty-two-year-old—soon to graduate and embark on life's journey, not exactly sure of his next step when he's out on his own. But Dan is sixty-four, and art is not his profession but his passion. He is also a retiree who spent thirty years as a medical doctor—an ophthalmologist to be precise.

I was particularly interested in meeting with Dan when I heard that he'd left his successful career practicing medicine only to begin all over again as a lowly freshman in a demanding art school in San Francisco. As soon as I met him, I realized that my image of him as a budding artist was totally a figment of my imagination. When he greeted me outside his front door, he appeared nothing like the bohemian version in my head, which was that of a man slightly disheveled with long, stringy dark hair, at least a couple day's worth of facial stubble, and maybe an earring.

Dan stood medium height. He was clean-shaven and gray-haired around the edges of his mostly-balding head. A warm, engaging smile lit up his face that was framed with contemporary black-rimmed glasses. Dressed in a blue-checked sport shirt and jeans, he was hardly the brooding artist I was prepared to encounter. So much for stereotypes!

As the only full-time college student in my study, I hoped his experience would inform me in ways I could pass along to you. In fact, I learned quite a bit from him. But first, I want to share something about the environment in which he lives and creates art.

If there is any pattern to the lifestyles of the artists I've interviewed, it's the remoteness of their homes and the difficulties posed to me in finding them! I suggested that Dan and I meet at his home rather than the Academy of Art University in San Francisco, since his home studio would reflect the art student and allow me to actually see his tarp-covered living room strewn with easels and paints. But I didn't realize that he lived off a private road in an enclave originally owned by the Jesuit Brothers and now shared with a Jesuit Retreat Center. So I wasn't sure I was outside of his house, nestled in some woody hills in northern California, until he appeared outside of his door, talking on his cell phone to a confused, somewhat embarrassed interviewer who thought she was lost.

We stepped inside, and the whitewashed interior was bright with natural light streaming through oversized windows into a very modern interior. This was particularly surprising on a cold winter day with an only-lukewarm sun low in the sky.

Every surface was covered with visual delights: paintings on the wall, sculptured busts on glass shelves, on pedestals, even on the piano, and studies of face parts, like bronze noses and lips of various sizes and shapes, hidden behind the sofa on a small tarp. Canvases too large to hang, and too many to make hanging possible, were stacked against a wall—most were works in progress, class studies, or homework assignments.

Dan's environment didn't always look like an art gallery. Prior to four years ago, he was an appreciator of art—someone who would go to the art museums and galleries, just like most of us do, to spend some enjoyable moments recharging dull senses after a nonstop week. But a few months before he turned sixty, something happened that changed his life dramatically.

"I was getting ready to retire and I said, 'Oh my gosh, what am I going to do? I'll have all this time on my hands.' I used to like art. I would go to all these art shows. I received an invitation to this woman's gallery exhibit, so I got out of surgery early that day and I thought, 'I'm going to go up to the city just to see what this is like.' When I got up there, it was really cool."

Not expecting more than an enjoyable evening, he went to this particular art exhibit opening because he had the time and a personal invitation. He reasoned that even if the art wasn't good, the wine, interesting conversations, and the possibility of live music would deliver a fine experience. Dan went alone. He is comfortable doing things this way; he is a single man.

In speaking with one of the artists whose very geometric and precise paintings caught Dan's attention, he learned that the artist taught in an art school in San Francisco, and Dan was encouraged to take one of his classes. Curious to learn more, he took a tour of the school, which was having its annual art show at the time. "I walked in and my mouth dropped. If I could do this after four years, sign me up!" He also fell in love with a student's painting, which he bought and used for inspiration. "I look at it every single day and say, 'Yup, that's what I'm striving to do.'"

And that was the beginning of Dan's artistry—as simple as that. The college signed him up, and he recalled his earliest experience. "My first day of class, I'm in this classroom with a whole bunch of kids just in their first semester out of high school. Talk about weird." He laughed heartily as he glanced back in time. "This was a charcoal drawing class, and there were drawings by kids from previous years up on the wall. I thought, 'My God, I will never in my wildest dreams—I could work for a hundred years, and I could never make anything like that.' And sure enough, at the end of the semester, I had something that I was pretty proud of." By the time he finished telling this story he all but jumped out of his seat to emphasize his amazement. "I could barely draw stick figures, but it's a skill they teach you."

As I listened, it sounded like becoming a serious art student was an instant good choice. But Dan had his doubts. "These kids have been drawing since they were six years old. They are the ones who go to art school, and I had never done anything like that before, so they were all so much better than me."

We talked about talent and whether or not it's necessary, but Dan's focus was squarely placed on interest and being pleased by the experience rather than being good. Considering talent, he concluded that you may have it or you may not, but it really doesn't matter. He added, "You don't have to have talent, you just have to put in the time." And, I suggested, you need the necessary capacity to persevere, to keep going even when discouraged, which is a characteristic of the Vintage Years that is easier to come by at that stage of life. "I'll sit down at a blank canvas and know what I want to paint, or I'll have a picture and I'll look at it for fifteen minutes and say, 'Oh my God, I'm never going to be able to do that.' And then, when I finally get started, it looks terrible. But when I get about ninety percent through it, I say, 'Oh, this is starting to look okay,' and when I finish, 'Wow, that looks great!'"

Dan has quite an unconventional retirement. His life is now as busy as it's ever been. It may not be for everybody, but the point is that this choice was the right one for Dan. "It's a lot of work. I don't think I have any talent, but I think I can produce works of art that please me. I look at the kids in my class, and they're all so worried. They're going to have to sell their art. It's hard work to make a living at it. I have zero desire to sell right now, and I don't have to."

I commented that Dan's art is done to please himself, without the marketing problems that working artists encounter. He agreed but added that pleasing his friends is important, and he gives much of his art away. This is consistent with what other artists in my study reported and consistent with Vintage Years' behavior. This is the life stage in which *generativity* is most pronounced. You may recall Erikson's life stages from Chapter 3 and his concept that describes the tendency to give back, give forward, and make a difference in the world through your accomplishments, leaving a legacy of sorts. "I could give some of these pieces to my nieces and nephews, and I guess it is something for them to think about me and remember me by." But he laughingly admits that they aren't all necessarily interested.

Digging around for even more clues to help explain Dan's trajectory into the arts, I wondered aloud about any other life experiences that might have contributed to his choice of fine arts. Did his mother love post-Impressionist art? Did he have an artsy counselor in summer camp or a mentor in a high school art class? The answer was a resounding no to all. But then he remembered an experience.

"Maybe ten or fifteen years before I retired, I went to Italy with a friend. We were in the Peggy Guggenheim museum. There was a canvas painted white, and they had taken a knife and made three vertical slash marks in it. I looked at that and said, 'I can do that.' And my friend looked at me and said, 'Then why don't you?' So I was thinking about it, and thinking about it. It seemed simple enough that even I could do it." When Dan returned from Italy, he tried to do an abstract painting; he actually did it, and pointed to the spot on the wall where it was proudly hung. At that time, he was about fifty. Life kept him sufficiently distracted for another ten years, but the incubation process had already begun.

Being the psychologist that I am, I felt a need to pursue the subject of his early life in more detail, especially regarding formative experiences that could have predicted Dan's current interests. Noting his French last name, I wondered if he had some Impressionist ancestors. Not exactly. His dad's family came from the Loire valley, an ancient region in central France known for its gardens and vineyards. They were all musicians—which is, after all, an art form.

Dan's great-great-grandfather was a blind musician and composer who traveled through Cuba and the Caribbean playing organ music in churches before eventually settling in Baton Rouge, Louisiana. The music stopped, Dan laughingly recalled, with his grandfather, who was a piano tuner. His physician father was a general practitioner and surgeon, who did house calls and kept very long hours but "played an awful violin, which he would torture us with sometimes." While Dan and his five siblings, of which he is the eldest, played musical instruments as children, "None of us was willing to put in the time."

Sensing I had reached a dead end in soliciting any additional information about family influences, we toured Dan's home gallery and garage where copious school projects were catalogued. With my help in balancing piles, we carefully moved envelope-sized to almost-life-sized works on canvases to get to his class studies and works in progress. I was the willing recipient of his mini lectures and actually learned quite a bit.

His self-portrait, a bust in bronze, was sitting next to another bust that at first glance seemed identical. He reminded me of the golden ratio that I vaguely remembered from a college art appreciation course long ago. The golden ratio depicts the relative scale of the human body, as well as everything else, including buildings, it turns out.

Based on a Greek mathematician's calculations about multiples of the number 1.618, it is otherwise known as phi. When applied to anatomy, the formula is called the Divine Proportion, and there is actually an ideal face, which is considered the face of beauty.

When Dan applied the golden ratio to his own face, the proportions of the second bronze head were slightly different and, according to him, better looking than he actually is in person. I could see what he meant. Our perception of physical beauty is hardwired and based on how closely one's features reflect phi in their proportions. The closer the fit, the more attractive the appearance seems to us.

I guess this is the sort of thing you learn in a four-year art program which, for Dan, will soon be coming to an end. To that point, Dan is a bit nervous realizing that without structure and deadlines, he's not sure how he'll manage his time. That remains to be seen. No sooner did he voice his concern than he happily noted that since bronze sculpting is his favorite art form, and with plans to take a course in that medium shortly after graduation, his worries will not likely materialize.

9 Darya: Mixed Media Artist

The Redwood City Art Center is home to thirty-four artists who work in a spectrum of media including painting, photography, drawing, jewelry design, Chinese calligraphy, and mixed media. This busy co-op houses their studios in a two-story, ten-thousand-square-foot boxy building resembling a motel. Various sized studios sit adjacent to each other along long carpeted corridors. However, unlike any motel I've ever seen, the wall space between studios was totally lined with art—large murals painted in vivid colors. This is the environment where new and seasoned artists rent space to create and showcase their art. This is where I met with Darya.

Wearing a parka covering multiple layers to ward off the January chill, even in the building, Darya, a colorful figure no taller than five feet, guided me through the maze-like setting, greeted along the way by an assortment of welcomes emanating from various open doors as we passed. Finally at her studio, probably no bigger than ten feet square, I quickly took a chair beside the portable radiator.

While a wooden table held a few books, all of the art materials were strewn about on the floor: canvasses, brushes in a cup, a roll of paper towels, fabric, pastels, paints, and jars with lids, contents unknown. She was quick to explain that she works on the floor and with the studio in this kind of array; she didn't want to clean the place up and give me the wrong impression.

At sixty-two, Darya is petite but strong, intense in her style and very self-determined. She spoke in a low, almost hushed tone, as if something she said shouldn't be overheard. Slowly and thoughtfully, she weighed each word and seemingly re-flected on it as it flowed out. I wondered if this was a personal characteristic or honed by thirty years of practicing law and be-ing a litigator, the kind of lawyer who builds and presents cases in court.

It turns out that her lawyering years, now in the past, were bittersweet. While she felt good about her ability to do the work and represent her clients well, she claims to have never wanted to be a lawyer. "I hated it the first day. I hated it the last day. I hated it every day in between." So, at fifty-eight, she finally closed her office for good. I commented that while her pragmatic side resonated with her work, her aesthetic side went begging. She seconded the statement: "Bingo, you got that exactly right."

Her decision to close her office followed a horrendous year in which her husband, sister, and mother died. Reeling from the losses and overwhelmed with handling multiple estates, she re-treated inward to recover and regroup. This also became a time for reflection, looking back at her life for cues about the next stage that she felt forced to live. "I felt that the rest of my life was going to be hell, because at that moment, it was hell. My heart was broken, my soul was broken, my brain was broken. But I said to myself, you live your life, whatever it is."

Darya was born in Salt Lake City, the youngest of three daughters. Her idol was always her next older sister, ten years her senior, who could do anything. At a very young age, Darya concluded that her sister "was the family artist and that I should do something else, maybe with an intent to individuate myself, I don't know. Certainly, nobody dissuaded or discouraged me in any way." As she mentioned her belief that she wasn't and couldn't be artistic, a belief she carried until very recently, I could readily see how she needed to find a unique path, as the youngest of three girls, in order to stand out. Her sister took the artist-child position even before Darya was born. This reflects the typical family dynamics in which the firstborn carves a niche in the family that subsequent siblings generally avoid. Darya needed to find another route in order to stand out.

Reflecting on her earliest years as anything but an artist, her exposure to art was indeed limited. "Other than crayons and painting, primarily in school, that was about it. Except, I remember as a child I was absolutely obsessed with color. I just loved color, and if I had blocks or if I had boondoggle—a thin plastic rope that you braid and make key chains or lanyards—I put the colors together. The black with the red . . . and I had these strong, strong feelings."

She went on to describe other color combinations that evoked immensely strong feelings. "My sister and I both had what I believe is called synesthesia, a very strong association of letters of the alphabet with colors. Sometimes they would migrate, but E is always red, N is always blue, and Y is always white. I would spend hours learning them. As soon as I started looking at letters of the alphabet, I associated them with colors."

I had personally never encountered anyone with synesthesia, a neurologic process that affects cognition and perception, seems to run in families, and is not all that uncommon. Some individuals with this condition know they have it, and others are more or less oblivious or just take it for granted. Synesthetic perceptions can vary in intensity, as Darya described, and tend to aid the creative process. This would seem to be an advantage to an artistic child like Darya.

Perhaps as a result of the hours putting blocks together or playing school with her older sister in the afternoons, kindergarten was utterly boring because she could read and tell time by then. By second grade, her teachers were praising her academic ability, not her artistry, and "that's when I shifted my attention away from any arts into educational pursuits." Darya's choice was not unusual for most children—they follow praise from the outside world when their inner drive is lukewarm. It's the path of least resistance!

Excelling at foreign languages and English, Darya buried her artistic potential for the next fifty years. This pattern is a common one, clearly borne out by the literature on child and adult development and the experience of others in my study. When a child is not exceedingly confident or identified as a gifted artist, and their ability isn't reinforced by others like teachers and parents, they find the arts are just too difficult to pursue in addition to the demands of adolescence and adulthood.

After college, a temporary job as a legal secretary led to Darya's dubious decision to attend law school. This was a pragmatic choice, consistent with her intellectual abilities and promising a decent salary and lifestyle but lacking the passion she so early in life associated with color and making things with her hands. The die was cast, and her adulthood was spent achieving in her profession and later finding a partner, making a home, and enjoying the visual arts as a spectator.

She recalled her student days in New York. "When I wasn't in class, I was always at museums, especially the Whitney. I don't know why, but the museum just did it for me, and some of the abstract artists—especially from the early 50s, the post-war abstract artists—just knocked me flat," she exclaimed with her intense but whispered passion. "I always had that interest in the visual arts."

One such occasion stands out in her mind as pivotal in her later return to the arts. A traveling exhibit came to town when Darya was in her late forties. "I think it was called the 'Whitney on Wheels.' I walked in and I saw across the gallery. I saw an Adolph Gottlieb painting that I remembered from when I was in college, and I stood there and just sobbed. Clearly visual arts have always affected me deeply." She recalled the feeling, gave a little shudder as if she was still there, and noted it was like seeing an old friend.

Time marched on, and Darya continued to visit museums when she could, enjoying the experience but still convinced that artistic talent eluded her. She dabbled in quilting, knitting, embroidering, sewing, and other crafts along the way, "always using bright colors." This was her way to relax and use her hands in creative ways. It may also have served as an interim diversion only obvious in retrospect. As a high-achieving person, I'm guessing she could not imagine doing art as long as she believed she couldn't excel. What changed that made it possible for her to take her first art class at fifty-eight?

Following her long-standing interest in quilting, she took it to the next level doing what is called art quilting, requiring an artist's perspective regarding texture, color, and design. Still not thinking about this as art but as a craft, she said resolutely, "I can do this," and set out to do fabric art at fifty. Quite by accident, she found a class by talking to an experienced quilting instructor. Darya recalled excitedly, "It all seemed very familiar to me: the cloth, the colors, the shapes, the tools." Later, while attending a quilting show, she was amazed. "These were not things you put on your bed. These were works of art." Still protesting the existence of her inner artist, she insisted, "But art quilting is not for me. I'm not an artist."

When Darya was getting ready to finally close her practice at fifty-eight, she "saw this little flyer. A lady in this very building was giving art classes: all styles; all levels; blah, blah, blah. I'm going to do this. I have no talent, but I'm going to see. I'm going to let a professional tell me I have no talent. I fell in love with pastels; I just went berserk for pastels because there is physicality with them. You can touch them and you apply them directly," she exclaimed, recalling her love of the tools and the hands-on experience. "One of the first pastels I ever did, my teacher said was wonderful and that I should put it in the county fair."

"I still don't believe that I have any native talent," she adamantly admitted, "but I don't care!" We both laughed as we realized this is one of the hallmarks of the Vintage Years.

Bringing the conversation to the present moment, she said, "Everyone here is very supportive and I'm truly enjoying it. I still love pastels, but I went into acrylics. I tried to integrate my interest in fiber art with fine arts." She pointed to a piece of upholstery fabric she was building on with paints and bits of metal screen. She pointed to another with "fabric on the back, paper glued on, there's paint, there's oil pastel, here's metallic string. I'm going to glue this down." I asked what she called this type of art, admitting my ignorance. "Mixed media, with fiber and paint. I'm sixty-two years old and I'm at the place where '[if you] tell me you can't do this, you can't put copper screen on top of fabric,' give it your best shot, buddy," she protested to an imaginary critic. I was impressed by her feisty defense of the artist within whom she now recognizes and holds dear.

Wondering what it would have been like to go to art school at twenty, she quickly realized that "if someone said at that time, 'You can't do that! Excuse me young lady, that's not allowed!' I might have believed them." So it appears that timing is a critical dimension and caring mightily about what others think is thankfully dialed way down in the Vintage Years.

Darya gestured to the floor where she usually sits surrounded by an array of art materials. "I realize that much of art, for me anyway, has to come out of chaos. You start in the middle. You have no idea where you are going. With me, the chaos of art, making a mess on the floor, knocking a paint can over, and ruining a canvas—the chaos is how art is made, and letting myself be chaotic is my current project. Just letting it happen is what I try to do now."

Having covered the four windows of her office with her own fiber art to remove distractions, she prefers working here rather than home as there's no laundry and dishes to do—no other distractions. "I love to cocoon. I'm alone with my art. Sometimes, I even turn the lights off and just sit in the dark, and I watch the colors go by." What a wonderful image!

Beginning to wrap up, I realized that my enchantment with the interview may have cost me a parking ticket for an expired meter. Darya added one more bit of philosophy: "Life, even at its worst, is absolutely astonishing. I would like to think of myself as a witness to the fact that life is astonishing." She repeated this with her characteristic breathy passion, as she surveyed her studio filled with vivid colors, tactile shapes, and awesome chaos.

10 Mort: Mixed Media, Large Installations

Stories about his oversized works of art preceded our meeting, so when Mort answered the door, I was surprised to see a jockey-sized fellow, small and wiry, with a wry smile and a droll sense of humor. For example, the foot mat outside his front door read, "Go Away" instead of the traditional "Welcome." At eighty-six, he looked remarkably fit even though he shuffled a bit as he walked me toward his living room. His mind, as I would learn over the course of an hour, was as sharp as a tack.

Mort shares his modern, loft-style duplex with his art: large installments that defy labeling. To describe them as textured or multidimensional doesn't do them justice. A four-by-four-foot photograph of a baby's face hangs between the loft and the first floor. Mort said it was his grandchild's face. From her broad forehead, three objects extend out as if floating in space. He explained, "These are what she is thinking about." A milk bottle on the right and a toy on the left flank a fluffy white lamb in the center. They look like animated thoughts in a comic strip the way they project from the huge photo.

He laughed as he talked about his non-conventional style. I could imagine some of his works hanging in the Museum of Modern Art—they seem good enough to me. He denied that he is a real artist because, "I don't sell things and I don't do portraits." I suggested that his definition is too narrow, that he does his art out of interest, love, passion, and creativity. He contemplated then accepted and appreciated the broadened definition.

While Mort denied his status as an artist, he said he always suspected he could paint and draw, since he entertained himself that way as a child. His father was a housepainter who, according to Mort, could draw quite well. His older brother was sent to art school, maybe to pursue the art career that his father needed to sublimate in order to support a family. But his older brother wound up painting houses anyway. His practical family did not support or nurture Mort's other childhood interests: acting and singing. They steered him in a more serious direction—going to the university and becoming a chemist. "I also wanted to do something different," he said.

Whether accidental or serendipitous, all of his jobs working as a chemist involved color, so significant to a would-be artist. First came the metallurgy plant that made costume jewelry. Then came a company that manufactured paints, crayons, and colored pencils. Finally, Mort worked as a color chemist in a patterned wallpaper plant where color needed to be managed so that a flower was distinguishable from its border. Mort's career as a color chemist was closely related to art, but the artist in him never found artistic expression in his job. We discussed the irony of his so-close-yet-so-far situation, and he remarked that his hands were full raising children, providing for them, working, commuting, and having time for his wife who died twelve years ago.

At sixty-one, a few years before retirement, Mort and his wife moved to the gated, over-fifty-five community on the east coast where he still lives and where he began his art hobby. Shortly after arriving, he attended a community art exhibit and saw some paintings that inspired him. He said to himself, "I can do better." He reported this to me with a sly smile, recognizing how grandiose it must have sounded given his lack of training and experience. He signed up to take some classes at the local community college. The rest is history!

Mort said, "I never really feel right unless I'm painting something. I'm edgy and agitated unless I'm working on a painting." "What does painting do for you?" I asked. "I love the adulation of others' responses to my work. I've got to have it, that's just the way I am," he replied. I suggested that part of what drives his artwork is his thought, "Wait until others see this!" This ham, who would have loved to be an actor, agreed wholeheartedly that he loves applause for his performance!

We talked briefly about how the brain functions and whether his art is useful in keeping his brain firing optimally. He nearly popped out of his seat at that point: "Definitely! Definitely, I feel smarter, intuitively smarter, and sharper when I'm doing art." Regarding his physical well-being, he noted, "I think the art helps. I'm tired when I'm not painting. I say, 'I think I need a nap, because I'm not working on stuff.' Also, I like painting. People know me by that. It leads to conversation. People ask, 'Are you working on anything?' I like that. It makes me feel good."

Mort took me for a tour, and I saw humor in the details he paints—like the family dinner with food on the floor under the child's chair, the red wine stain on the table cloth next to the wine decanter, and the dog begging for crumbs with his front paws on the table. He captured the tumult of an extended-family meal with all of its idiosyncrasies, and it made me laugh. Mort enjoyed watching me—an audience of one.

He pointed out that he used more red color in the base and green color in the top to create the optical illusion that the painting is moving forward at the bottom and receding at the top. He explained that his chemist's brain was at work here: those colors create an illusion of near and far. This was news to me, but I could see what he described.

The *coup de grace*, as far as I am concerned, is his "New Year's Eve on Broadway" painting, showing the dynamic shapes of that place, the events, and a sea of people suspended from the canvas to provide the three-dimensional aspect. In the middle of his painting is a slit with a paper digital clock inserted, displaying twelve-midnight. His humor was again at play when he suspended this five-by-five-foot painting in the cutout between his kitchen and living room and inserted a real digital clock where the paper one had been. At midnight, his New Year's Eve guests got to see the clock strike twelve o'clock in real time. This was the ultimate dynamic painting! I viewed the rest of his art: typically quirky, humorous, edgy, and imbued with the passion and energy that Mort swears keeps him alert and vital.

When I looked over the short questionnaire Mort filled out, in answer to my question, "How has the practice of your art form changed your life?" he wrote, "My life is more exciting—people know me." Mort the would-be actor and singer, now painter, finally has an appreciative audience.

7 Writers

Long before written symbols existed, all kinds of ideas were communicated verbally. The knowledge of a generation was transmitted to the next in the form of compelling stories which captured the interest and attention of the listeners, who needed to remember them for subsequent generations. All matters of daily life benefited from this oral tradition. Anything that was tried and proven true would become a legend. No point in metaphorically reinventing the wheel!

And then came the written word, ushering in much less distortion and more accuracy of information. Storytelling, once a necessity, could now become an art form, a way of communicating much more than the facts of life. As long as people have been able to read and write, they had the capability to creatively write stories, but most don't until their Vintage Years.

Go to any senior citizens' center today, and there's a good chance that it offers a memoir-writing group. Why is that? Our elders have something to say, and for all the reasons cited in Part

I, they wait to do it until this later life stage. Some find they have talent, which is both surprising and delightful. Some enjoy the process of sharing their wisdom based on a lifetime of experience. Still others want to leave a legacy in the form of their personal or family history. But one fact is ubiquitous for all I spoke with: they feel energy, passion, and satisfaction when they write. It's fun. Plus, at this point in life, writing is both the process and the outcome—no longer do the storytellers feel a need for any kind of externally driven goal or reward.

Seven writers will share their adventures on the following pages.

1 Kathleen: Poetry and Non-fiction Writer

Kathleen's home is on the other side of what looks like a secret passage through an opening in a ten-foot hedge. I found a weathered wooden gate beyond which I could see a house surrounded by so much greenery that it looked like a cottage in the middle of a forest rather than on a busy street corner. Walking through the person-sized opening felt like going into a magical space. The glass-enclosed French doors closest to where I stood suggested a living room, not the front entrance, except for the dead-bolt lock half way up the frame. Kathleen greeted me at the door, which was indeed the front entrance of the house. It led directly into the modest-sized living room where we greeted each other and looked for a place to sit.

Kathleen towered over my five-foot-three-inch frame. She has short, wavy gray hair that she wore casual and free flowing, like the aging hippie I imagined her to be. I thought about how she might have looked forty years ago—with long, thick, wavy hair blowing in the breeze and wearing a tie-dyed long skirt and sandals. Steering myself back to reality, I noticed her sleeveless tan blouse covered with brown Chinese characters partially buttoned over a tank top. I handed her a short questionnaire. She glanced briefly at it, holding her pen, and began to talk unprompted by me. While periodically looking down at the sheet of paper, Kathleen seemed to view it as an interruption in her flow of words.

We spoke for nearly two hours, and though at first I tried writing furiously to take notes, I gave up, choosing instead to attend fully to her fascinating story. I had to trust that my smart phone voice-recorder was working properly. Fortunately, it was!

Kathleen believes that being creative—singing and making art—is hardwired into people but that it's not easy to reach our potential in the first part of life. "There's the issue of having to make a living for forty years, and then it's time to do something else." Only now that her school-teaching days are behind her can she actually take the time to reflect. "I've had many experiences that I didn't have time to think about before, but now I want to take time to understand them, and making a story about them helps me a lot." I asked her how, and she said, "I'm making meaning out of these random experiences. I'm looking for themes that underlie my entire life, I'm looking for patterns that explain who I am. There are a few things I would like to figure out, and writing seems to be a good way to do it. I don't think I'm unique, but if I can tell my story well, craft it, and hook it to some theme in my life, it will be somebody else's story, too."

She went on with her story. "I guess it might have been a day dream; I thought if I had the ability, the talent, I would be a writer. But I knew when I retired I would have to put that to rest, forget it, or do it!" she said, greatly emphasizing the last three words. "Just see what it would be like to take some writing classes." She was sixty-three, gearing up for her new life and thinking, "I will do a few things. I'm going to take oil painting, I'm going to write, I'm going to exercise more, I'm going to go to the gym, I'm going to hike—all those things. I'm going to sing." She went on without taking a breath, "I started singing the last year I worked. I said to myself, 'let's see if I can start this and then carry it through,' and so far, I have." She had taken a choir course in college, enjoyed it very much, but couldn't figure out how to integrate it into her busy life, so her singing was lost for decades.

"When I retired, I waited nine months or so before signing up for a writing class. For me, it was a high-risk thing to do, because I was going to read to others something I had written. I wasn't confident in my writing skills, and I didn't know how it would be to go personal in this memoir class, how it would feel to put very personal material out there. I've continued in the class ever since." I noted that this was about four years ago. "Now I also attend two writing critique groups." I wondered if once she had finished one class, it fanned the fire of her interest and caused her to stretch herself into other similar experiences. She agreed and then expanded on the idea in terms of connection to a community of like-minded seniors who give her feedback and listening power.

This group of sixty-to-ninety-year-olds has become very important to Kathleen. She looks forward to seeing them and hearing about their work on a weekly basis. They don't talk about their outside lives, but they share intimacy during the time they're together. "I get a lot of feedback. It's positive. It's just a senior center, but it's nice," she laughs. "I have a way of saying things," she trailed off as she realized she sounded boastful. This was her newfound confidence speaking.

One unexpected consequence of her writing is that Kathleen has corresponded with a few of her favorite authors. She took a chance on writing to them and sending a few lines of her own work, and they responded. She was amazed and flattered by their attention and observations—no one had ever commented on her writing when she was a child. Speaking of which, she remembered the story about a horse that she wrote when she was eight as she sat in bed on a rainy day. That was it for childhood writing.

"I don't mind spending a week writing eight hundred words. I'm slow, but I have the time now." She writes some things only for herself and to share with her classmates; these pages are generally about her family. Then she shreds them. She described this as therapeutic. "One piece had to be out, or I couldn't write anything else. It's still a little hard for me to say I'm a writer. I write every day, and if I'm not writing, I'm reading other people's writing." To sharpen her craft, I suggested. "At the beginning, I told myself, 'no pressure, write when you can,' but then I found that I liked it. Today I carried my computer to two different meetings thinking, 'Maybe I'll have a chance to write.'" True to her intentions, Kathleen writes for four hours every morning.

"To write at all, I had to be willing to write badly. My first drafts were just terrible, and I had to give myself permission to do that. That permission felt good by itself, knowing that I wouldn't be Annie Dillard or anyone like that. I have no ambition to send anything to *The New Yorker*. But I have something to say, my way." Having said this, Kathleen confessed her desire to be published and to be paid for something she wrote, which happened for her last year.

After submitting her best piece to a literary magazine and expecting her first of many rejections, she was amazed when they agreed to publish it. Later, when she met the magazine's circulation manager and told him that she wrote the piece about having lunch with her ninety-four-year-old mother, he replied effusively, "Oh, my wife sobbed over that story!" Several of Kathleen's pieces subsequently found their way into publications, so she really is a writer, and a published one to boot. We laughed together about her commercial success, including getting pub-lished in the *AARP Bulletin* whose readership numbers more than eleven million.

Curious about her backstory, I inquired into her family histo-ry. She and her husband have a blended family of five children. Their last child recently left home, opening up some space and time. But, Kathleen's mother has had difficulties since Kathleen was fifteen requiring Kathleen's ongoing care. Ironically, these experiences also provide her much of the deep, intensely emo-tional material for her writing. "I wrote this piece called, 'I'm So Lucky,' which is what my mother is always saying, even though I don't think she's so lucky."

Kathleen went on to describe her mother's situation. "A lot of what I write is about my mother. That's a story I want told. She has a remarkable attitude considering all the losses she's suf-fered. My mother was in a car accident on the way to work when she was forty-five. She had a cerebral hemorrhage and has not walked, read, written, thought clearly, or remembered anything well since—for fifty-one years." The need to get her mother's story told is multi-faceted: it is somewhat therapeutic, it is a de-sire to tell what her mother can't, and it is a tribute to her mother's strength.

As we ended the interview, Kathleen volunteered, "I've nev-er been happier. This is the happiest I've ever been." She told me about a piece she's written called "Why I Write." As she read it to me, I was struck by its poignancy, imagery, and relevance to this book. She was willing to let me share it with you and it ap-pears in the Appendix with a sampling of other artists' work.

2   Stan: Fiction Writer

Stan, at sixty-nine, is the picture of good health. Lean and muscular, he sat next to his bicycle helmet at the outdoor table at Starbucks wearing dark glasses, a red zip-up sweat jacket, and a baseball cap. When he's not writing, you might find him mountain biking or hiking. He's a retired medical doctor who practices the good health that he once preached.

One of the first things I learned about him was that, ironically, as a young student his most difficult subject was English. "I never thought I would be doing anything with English, period. I think that's what led me into the sciences; it let me do something which was easier for me." After a long career as a physician, he is writing novels. Not that this happened right away.

When he first started out as an allergist, he was the new doc on the block. He looked for a way to distinguish himself and stand out from the other allergists in the neighborhood. He started writing information that dispelled the myths about allergies and, over time, turned his offerings into a book, which he then gave to his new patients. "Quite a good marketing strategy," he noted, and I agreed.

More than a decade later, while recuperating from a neck injury incurred from clutching a violin too tightly as a beginning player, he lay in bed and wondered, "Can I write the end of a story at the beginning and keep people's interest until the end? Can I give them the answer to who did what to whom, but then keep the action and the plot going?" And so began his flirtation with the idea of writing novels, which grew during a time without structure—a new experience for him—as his recuperation dragged on. Stan's violin career ended abruptly, but his writing took off. He was almost sixty at the time.

One of the dilemmas he encountered was whether to shoot for writing a best seller or to write what he wanted for himself. The latter choice won out. Weighing the options, consistent with his analytic style, he ultimately rejected the idea of a commercial approach, because "If others don't like it, that's okay." He preferred to remain independent from those who would want to change what he wrote or put time constraints on its completion. In the Vintage Years, the goal is often no more than the pleasure of doing, without concern for societally bestowed benefits like fame and fortune.

"Fiction writing is fun. I can create people and I can get them to do what I want them to do." He joked that he's a bit controlling, but writing for fun lets him be in charge, which is important to him after decades of doing what may have been necessary to meet others' demands, standards, or time constraints. "There are still musts, but now I can choose when I do them," he quipped.

Regarding his writing style, Stan is totally self-taught. "I can see myself in some of the output. It's not biographical," he assured me, "but the style, and the phrasing is not what you would learn in a writing class. I've never taken a writing class, so I don't know for sure, but I doubt that it is." His need to do things alone and in his own way won out over any need for a writer's community or instruction. As an introvert, Stan is comfortable and content to spend time by himself and heed his own counsel.

Our conversation went off on a tangent when Stan brought up the questions long pondered by philosophers. "The brain is a total mystery to me. Where do ideas come from? The brain is a bunch of neurons. How does an organic chemical come up with a thought?" There is no short answer, of course, and a lengthy one based on neuropsychological research findings didn't seem to fit in the context of a noisy outdoor cafe. Stan's face showed skepticism as we talked about the way the brain might facilitate the artistic endeavors of an older person. He couldn't agree that aging itself informed his writing in any particular way.

Returning to our interview, Stan described his current project: "It takes the Moses story and transplants it into nineteenth-century Russia. I found historical incidents in Russia that would correlate with the Bible. It's fictional history, I guess you could call it, but it's not historical fiction, which is actual events taking place with fictional characters inserted into the actual events along with the real-life characters. In my story, everybody is fictional, pretty much." Satisfied with this distinction, his body straightens up as he proudly announces, "There's prose, and to represent biblical times, poetic style—and I'm not a poet." He sounds a bit surprised by his revelation, as if reminding the kid from long ago that English is indeed manageable.

His skepticism took another turn when he suggested that although older people have more time, it often gets spent on their health problems or on caring for spouses, like his wife who suffered two serious health problems in as many years. "The emotional demand, financial demands, and other stuff that goes on; that needs to be compartmentalized if you are going to do anything else. It takes time." Sensing the conversation might be turning a bit too personal, I changed direction and focused instead on ways to use art to distract from unpleasant thoughts or situations. "That's been true for me. When I'm at the computer and focused, everything else is in the background. I don't do this to get away from something, but it is distracting." He acknowledged that his laser-focused writing gives him some relief from the health problems in his family.

"I used to write very early in the morning. Somehow I stopped doing that and wrote later in the morning. Now, I don't have a set schedule. If the weather's nice, I might want to be outside rather than inside writing." Stan reiterates his disdain for having to do things a certain way. Ideas come when they do. When ideas come to Stan, he will stop and jot something down.

Referring to his current project, he said, "I wrote the whole thing out and then learned that you can't have a book that long, so I divided it up into five books. I was working on the first of the books, and that turned out too long, so I cut that in half. That book is all done and published." He quickly added, "It was self-published on an Internet site where you can do it for free. I have to buy a book to get a copy, just like anybody else." His current plan includes finding an agent and promoting his book. But, he confesses that he puts very little time into doing so, as it's not his primary interest. "The minute I decided to write it for me, the way I wanted it, which is unconventional because I haven't seen a book put together like this, I said, 'I like reading it, it's printed, here's a copy, it's good enough for me.'"

And so our time came to an end. As we parted, I was sure that Stan would finish the rest of the novels in his series, have them printed and bound, and enjoy them in the same way.

3 Michelle: Novelist

If ever a place inspired writing, this was it. My journey began in a fog-encased paradise one August morning in the Santa Cruz Mountains. This was where I met and interviewed Michelle, a former bankruptcy attorney, who took down her shingle to write a novel.

After turning off Highway 1, the old road that skirts the Pacific Ocean and stretches north to south from one tip of California to the other, I was enveloped in trees. The fog and dew in this densely wooded area mingled to cloud my windshield and got me to turn on my headlights although it was barely ten in the morning.

Another few minutes passed as I drove on a country road that finally opened into a clearing where I saw a house dwarfed and encircled by redwood trees so tall that the fog shrouded their tops. This is where Michelle lives, having moved here from the north Silicon Valley city of Palo Alto.

The etched-glass front door of her home opened into a huge front room rimmed completely on two sides by floor-to-ceiling windows and a huge stone fireplace. Michelle was dressed in warm sweat clothes covering the kind of body that practices yoga and takes hikes. In her decisive, take-charge style, she ushered me in, offered a seat by the oversized window, and put the tea kettle on the stove.

After thirty years of practicing law, raising two kids, and managing a household, Michelle was open to some kind of change. The timing worked well, since her husband had just taken a voluntary work transfer. The decision to move into the heart of nature was a big one for these urban folks originally from New York City. I wondered whether living in paradise led to writing or whether Michelle's itch to write led to living in this remote but majestic place. Our interview couldn't resolve this chicken-egg conundrum.

Once they were settled in this small rural town, Michelle continued some of her legal work remotely for four years, but the desire to write the novel that was stuck in her head led to closing her law practice and focusing her energy entirely on writing. She was in her mid-fifties.

When I referred to her as a writer, she seemed surprised and squirmed a bit in her seat. Though she spends much of her day working on her novel, she doesn't consider herself a writer. She has no formal credentials or license as she does to practice law, and she did not want to seem an impostor. She simply writes. And write she does.

As we sipped tea in her comfortable and serene living room, I was struck by her patience and persistence as a writer who hasn't taken a writing course since her college days as an English major. She credited her discipline to her left-brain, problem-solving approach to most things. She laughed, recalling her engineer father, who wound up with three daughters of which she was the oldest. Whether she learned or inherited his linear style is hard to unravel, but it served her well in her chosen analytic profession.

Time changes our preferences. As Michelle approached her Vintage Years, curiosity began to bubble to the surface of her consciousness. Long-dormant and unexplored parts of herself began pushing for expression. The once-upon-a-time English major came back to life. "I have always read a lot. That's my thing. In the past, I tried to write a couple of times. I tried to write a mystery, but I had two small children. I spent all of my spare time thinking over the legal things I had done during the day." Her other attempt was during a one-year leave of absence. "I tried to write then, but there was just too much going on." Not surprising, Michelle's current attempt at writing coincided with the move to their new surroundings and the pastoral lifestyle that it provided.

The quiet, peaceful setting serves as a backdrop for her surging creativity. "When I moved here—it's so incredibly beautiful. If I was ever going to write, this was the place. If I couldn't do it here, I really couldn't do it, and I should realize that this wasn't the thing I was going to do." I commented that visually, it's like living in a still-life picture. She can sit and look through the window behind her computer monitor in the warm, earthy, wood-paneled, beam-ceilinged office that is spacious, sparse, and yet cozy. Here she can dream up her novel's characters and breathe life into them.

With most of her friends far away and no ready-made local community, Michelle is often alone with her thoughts, which appeals to her and fortunately fits with her solitary style. It wouldn't fit for everyone, but it definitely seemed appealing to me. Her daily pattern consists of waking up, dressing in sweats, spending time with her husband before he leaves for work, and then sitting down to write. Letting her creativity flow and envelope her in the inner world of her unfolding story distracts her from any other thoughts and transports her to another place and time, until she emerges to take a hike in the redwoods.

Not all of her days have been so tranquil. For nearly a year, she battled an illness that left her little time and energy for writing. But even then, she wrote when she could, and the act of writing seemed to have shielded her, though temporarily, from the worrisome process of her medical situation and an unknown outcome. Her experience is similar to the other artists I interviewed who can enter into their craft so fully that their pain and apprehensions take a time-out from their awareness for hours at a time.

Finally able to put her health concerns aside, Michelle resumed writing more consistently but now finds herself distracted after a half hour. Adapting to her current situation, Michelle uses breaks more often and then returns to writing. She reported this adjustment in her writing habit in a hushed voice, as if she was somehow slacking off.

A half hour without interruption seems a pretty good interval to me. Clearly, her standards and work ethic are high; they are matched by her passion for what she is doing and how she spends her time. "I have arthritis, so I take about four minutes in the morning to do stretching exercises. Then I go sit at my desk." I asked for details; the how and what that others might find useful for getting started on their own. "Every day, I put markers where I start working and where I finish. The next day, I reread what I wrote the day before, and that gets me back into exactly where I was."

At the end of a day of writing, which might be a couple of hours that produces a couple of pages, Michele described feeling "refreshed and invigorated." She then takes time for daily rituals that she enjoys, such as hiking, yoga, and chi gong.

She laughed about her progress as a writer. "I've been doing it for six years, working on this one novel. In the beginning, I thought, 'Well, I could go to school, and get a Master of Fine

Arts degree.' That's what a lot of people recommended. That wasn't what I wanted to do. I wanted to just sit and do what I wanted to do. If it took me longer, then that was fine. I wanted to stay here in this quiet and not participate in a program somewhere else. I made a lot of mistakes. What I'm writing now is not what I started writing six years ago, but it's been a fascinating learning process anyway."

As the interview drew to a close, Michelle confided that she had another story in mind that will likely be her next book. It had actually been her first idea when she started to write, but she put it aside in favor of what seemed easier at the time. Now, this writer who is not comfortable describing herself as such, has a second and even third book in mind—and a life of writing that will extend well into the future.

Though she couldn't answer my nagging research question about how her artistic practice enhances her physical, psychological, or cognitive well-being, she perceives that her life is infused with meaning and contentment. The Vintage Years have a pull of their own toward doing what is pleasurable, meaningful, and satisfying.

Michelle freely acknowledged her good fortune to spend her time this way and not have to maintain a job for financial reasons. She also realizes that her writing lifestyle could not have happened at an earlier point in her life when time was scarce and external goals required her attention. "I was not at all creative as a child, but I am now able to access that part of myself."

Michelle's self-reflection echoes what Jonah Lehrer points out in his book, *Imagine: How Creativity Works*. The relaxed mind contributes to the free flow of creative juices, according to Lehrer. "When our minds are at ease—when those alpha waves are ripping though the brain—we're most likely to direct the spotlight of attention *inward*, toward that stream of remote associations emanating from the right hemisphere."[24]

The alpha waves he mentioned are associated with wakeful relaxation; these are slower brain waves than those produced by the brain when it is engaged in focused activities that require full attention. Lehrer posits that in this relaxed state of mind, insights otherwise not available come to awareness. Michelle's current life, free at last from the daily need to laser-focus, is perfect for writing novels.

---

[24] p.31

4   Anne: Haiku and Local History Writer

Meeting with Anne was a wonderful bonus. Her husband, Don the renaissance man whose story is also included in this book, suggested I talk with her about her passion since retirement—writing about local history.

Anne was dressed for the rugged, rural mountainside where she lives: jeans, tee shirt, and sturdy shoes, but also delicate earrings, revealing different parts of her complex character. She was welcoming and cheerful, which was greatly appreciated after my adrenaline-filled drive along the one lane road through the fog up Mt. Diablo. Surely Mt. Diablo, which means "thicket of the devil," was named for the threatening conditions I encountered.

Anne retired from a career as a high school English teacher when she was fifty-five, a couple of years after her husband stopped working. While she didn't say it, I wondered if her choice was influenced by his decision or whether the urge to write became too big to contain while she was working. Anne made it clear that as a teacher, mother of three kids, and woman of the house, she never had the time to pursue other interests to any extent. "When I was teaching high school English, there was no time for anything else: no time for quiet or creativity, except in the summer, and then you're recovering. And then, my creativity was focused on my teaching and making what they had to study next year interesting."

By definition, an English teacher is trained in writing, or at least with the skills to teach children how to write. Still, this is a long way from writing books and poetry, both of which have defined Anne's life for the past twenty years. In response to my question about how practicing her art form has changed her life, she gestured all around to the tables, bookcases, and cabinets that I could see and those that were beyond my view, saying, "There's clutter everywhere. There's stuff on the table in the sunroom. There's more material on the floor. If you go back there in the bedroom where the computer is, all over the bed there's more stuff." She laughed as we shared a knowing glance about the life of a nonfiction writer. She referred to the piles as clutter, but quickly laughed again and redefined it as "organizational materials everywhere." I understood fully, and appreciated her situation: she wrote two books simultaneously in one year and edited a book of haikus recently.

We returned to her story and her growing interest—for about twenty years now—in the road they've lived on for more than thirty years: Morgan Territory Road. Anne knew it had a history dating back well over a hundred years. In the more recently settled West, that's a significant amount of time. As she became increasingly curious, Anne realized that her investigation required more time than a high school teacher had to give. Her burning desire to learn more about the road and its early inhabitants provided the impetus to retire. She wondered, "Why did people move up here long ago? Probably not for the reason we did, that it was beautiful. And so I was curious about how it got settled. I began talking to people, and they would tell me about other people, who led me to still other people. That became my first book."

Anne summed up her first project all too quickly, making it seem easier than I knew it could have been. It took six years from beginning the research to finding a publisher with all the usual stumbling blocks "caused by editors who were unreliable in the struggle to find a publisher."

She read me the first sentence of the introduction about building their house, complete with an outhouse, while also living in it. "Toilet paper looped in the strong gusty wind like a Chinese kite as I stood shivering in the crisp morning air, balanced on the board that led to the portable outhouse." She read this sentence as if to an appreciative audience, which I was. I thought her sentence sounded more like poetry than prose. She said with some leftover indignation that her first editor thought it was the stupidest opening to a book that he ever read. Her later editor and publisher liked to boast about it. I was glad that she kept the courage of her convictions, something that's easier to do when you don't have to please anyone later in life.

"The San Francisco Public Library sent me a letter the other day," she declared. "They want three of my books." She beamed proudly. "My second book is also at the California Historical Society; it covers the history of the Livermore region."

It seemed to me that in order to write four books, and counting, a writer would have to be very disciplined and determined. I suspected that she approached her writing like her husband played the fiddle, every morning for two hours. But it was hard to pin Anne down. She writes when she feels like it, and certainly not for fame or fortune. "I write for myself. If you don't like what I wrote, you don't have to buy the book. You don't have to read it. I'm not trying to make money, so I'm not worried about who my audience is." I continued to be curious about when the actual writing takes place, so I pushed her for details.

Taking a minute to reflect on what she actually does, it seems that she writes when inspired, which turns out to be about three or four days a week. She likes mornings and late evenings—these are the times when she has the most energy. Interestingly, her husband plays the fiddle before she is awake in the morning, and she writes after he is asleep in the evening. "I have self-imposed deadlines," Anne volunteered.

We talked about one of the luxuries of the second half of life, when the need to make a living, or the desire to make one's mark on the world, or to be famous, or to compete takes a back seat to "This is what I want to do, period!" While she didn't report that writing was a legacy goal, one unforeseen consequence was that her son wrote a book, a biography about an early bicycle racer. "He said that it was my writing that inspired him." She stopped at this point, as if looking backward to that conversation with her son. A big smile of motherly pride swept over her face.

About poetry, she explained that it was an interest of hers many years ago. A year after her retirement, while visiting a friend and quite accidentally, the way lots of interests get started, she was introduced to haiku. "My friend had some books spread out and went to make some tea. I was looking at a book about haiku poetry. She told me about the Haiku Society and showed me their newsletter, and I said, 'I think I'd like to join this!'" A year later, Anne was a member of a regional group that spans about a hundred-mile radius, though Anne lived quite far from everyone else. Still, she made it to meetings periodically and then joined a second group that slightly overlapped the first geographically.

It happened just like that, the moment when she knew that something previously unknown became a driving force, so much so that in 2010, her volume of haiku poetry was published. This traditionally brief style of poetry consists of three phrases based on the number of syllables in each so that the first has five, the second seven, and the third five. Anne showed me a beautifully illustrated and designed book and read some of her haiku to me. Consider that haiku was new to Anne only fourteen years earlier! I asked her if I could include a couple in my book so that readers could better understand and appreciate the haiku form. She graciously agreed, and you'll find these haikus in the Appendix.

In response to my query about why she keeps writing she said, "There's that feeling of satisfaction, plus there's more to be said about local history." Some locals asked her if she could write a book about the history of the region, which turned into her second book, but she knew it would be an enormous undertaking. About that time she made a trip to Port Townsend, Washington, to see some friends who gave her a copy of a book about that place as a gift. She read the edited volume and thought she could do that—get a few people to share the writing.

Finding interested others proved to be difficult, and the only local resource never followed through with writing. "I ended up writing all of it. I had the time to do it. I've always been interested in books and libraries. When I was a little girl, one of my favorite places in the whole world was the local library. I love what my husband would say is ridiculous, tedious work," she said, referring to the research demands of writing nonfiction and sleuthing like Sherlock Holmes. "I guess I have the patience to see it through," she noted thoughtfully.

5 Caroline: Historical Memoirist

Caroline's stories kept me spellbound. Without a break between them and with such natural segue, I could hardly keep up with her or stop to ask questions while I furiously took notes. Wondering whether there was any way to capture her extraordinary ninety years and do it justice in a few pages, I resolved to listen and not worry about it. It was clear that this woman always had the makings of a writer, even if she didn't get free from responsibility until she was seventy-seven.

"Being New Englanders, I think storytelling was in everybody's bones, or maybe it was that period before TV when you got together on Sunday with the relatives. Everybody had a story to tell. I remember every night when my father came in the door, he always had something funny to tell. We were brought up always telling about our experiences, so when I went to college, I said to my mother, 'I can keep a journal or I can write to you in detail and you can keep the letters.' I had no idea then that I would end up in the army and have all these unusual things go on in my life."

Caroline's mother was also a writer; her book of poetry was published when she was 105! But her training was as a fine artist; she was awarded a bachelor's degree in art from the Pratt Institute in New York City in 1911, when women had few opportunities and could not yet vote. She served as a lifelong inspiration for her only daughter to take on anything she wished, which was borne out by Caroline's curiosity and adventuresome life.

Caroline was in college during World War II and studied nutrition. Having no background whatsoever in the arts, she simply wrote letters home every week, a tradition that began with her father who wrote daily letters to her mother during their ten-year courtship and his service during World War I. "I think I was always writing: I wrote on suitcases, I wrote in the bathroom, I wrote wherever I was. I was always writing home, probably two or three times a week. That probably gave me some background in writing. Phone calls were too expensive. Telegrams usually meant bad news. So that was how we kept in touch—writing. They were also writing to me. My father sent me a special-delivery letter every Sunday for four years. It cost fifteen cents, and the poor newsboy had to get on his bicycle and pedal from town all the way out to the campus."

It was 1944. No one knew how long the war might last. Every able-bodied person was prodded to do their fair share and patriotic duty. As resources stretched to the limit, the War Department reached out to Caroline's class of graduating nutrition students to serve in the armed forces. "Thinking, 'Why not?' I took the civil-servant exam, thinking it was just another class assignment. Six weeks later, I got a letter from the War Department." Caroline soon began a year of advanced training at Walter Reed Army Medical Center in Washington, DC. She earned her commission as a 2nd Lieutenant in the Army Medical Corps and served as a nutritionist at the hospital. She added that the document stipulated, "You will serve for the duration of the war. Well, in 1943, you didn't know what you were signing up for. But because the fella I was going with was one of the first people killed in the war, I thought I had to complete what he started."

This was the beginning of a "strenuous, challenging and fascinating" time for her. "Everyone came to Walter Reed. Mrs. Roosevelt came once a week to see her boys. I had the experience of taking care of General Pershing's and General Patton's meals. I was sent to San Antonio, Texas, for my basic training. Then, I was stationed in Memphis taking care of paraplegic patients. Three German prisoners of war worked in the ward kitchen. They were marvelous help. They would watch me do something—like making an omelet—only once, and then I never had to do it again."

There was no stopping Caroline! Between the stories she remembered off the top of her head and the ones memorialized in the weekly letters sent to her parents, it's easy to imagine how *Short Skirts and Snappy Salutes*, her first book published in 2004, came to be.

But how exactly did it come to be? Retracing her life in a glance: she survived her military days; she worked in the public sector in hospitals; she worked on a ship docked at a Manhattan pier on the East River serving poor, undernourished children; and later, she lectured on American antiques. Her husband's jobs took them across the eastern seaboard, the Midwest, the mountain states, and finally to California where she settled for good.

After caring for her mother for the last thirteen years of her long life, Caroline, at seventy-seven and a widow with two grown children, finally settled down after a lifetime of service. After grieving and sorting through her mother's effects, Caroline experienced the slowing down of time and pace that is familiar to most seniors. She wondered about her next steps and remembered the letters saved by her mother.

More than a half-century had passed since penning the letters, diligently saved by her mother and discovered when helping her move from the family home. Caroline reminisced about her surprise at finding such a gold mine of letters and post cards. "When she was leaving her house, when she was ninety-five, I went up in the attic. There was a trunkful, and then there were bags and boxes behind that.

"After I moved here, it took me a year to get them all lined up. I realized I had a wonderful record of the war, what I went through in the army, and what they went through on the home front. It was a very complete record. I started out to do this just for the family, and I took a course in memoir writing. The instructor thought it was too historic to be just for the family, this had to go further. But I didn't take that too seriously. I soon realized that I had to know how to use a computer, or I would never get all this done. So then I spent most of a year trying to get literate enough on the computer to go ahead." I queried about her age at the time; she was eighty.

Wondering about how she learned to navigate the computer from scratch, I wasn't really surprised to hear that she taught herself. Problem solving, surviving challenges, and persevering no matter what, had always served her well. It reminded me of her story about studying at night at the Walter Reed Army Hospital library after a day on the wards during her post-college training. Because she hadn't yet been commissioned as an officer, she was not allowed to sit in the library's reference room. So she stood the whole time at high study tables. What an amazingly adaptive and determined young woman!

Nudging Caroline back to the topic of how she mastered the computer, she volunteered, "I never took a course. My niece came out and bought me a computer and spent one afternoon telling me what I had to do." A friend she met in the memoir-writing class, who "was a whiz on the computer," helped her when she got stuck. "It takes an old brain a long time to take all this in. It was difficult."

I was quick to point out that an old brain is certainly capable of learning but that it does take longer and requires more persistence and review. A fair tradeoff is that as a senior, you have more time. Also, persistence is a hallmark of the Vintage Years. "Since mother lived to be 107, nothing surprises me about aging. I've seen it all before," she laughed. But Caroline, being a consummate storyteller, is off on a side tale about her mother's driving skill, or lack of it, at ninety-three.

Steering her back to the memoir class, which I thought readers would appreciate more; I wondered where she found the class to begin with and what she was looking for. It seems that one adult education class led to another. "I think the way to begin is not to think about writing a book but writing one incident at a time, and gradually you begin to accumulate a little knowledge and a little confidence. We had such a good time and learned the most from listening to each other read. The class met once a week for two and a half hours. The first two years, we were learning things, and the last two years, we were sitting next to each other just to read." She smiled broadly as she recalled her now good friend and fellow writer who was the computer guru. "The same group of people signed up again and again; we're almost like a family. You go through a lot with the people in the class. We all began to support each other."

When I questioned the need for the class beyond four years, Caroline was emphatic. "It's about the discipline. In the beginning, you need to have a class so that you do it. It means saying no to going to dinner or other things so that you do the writing, or it won't get done. That was an important part of it. You had to have the discipline, because you knew that next Tuesday you had a class and you needed to read."

Trying to further clarify and understand what discipline meant to her logistically, Caroline was very precise. "I never did get to the place where nine to twelve every day, I'm going to write. As the years have gone by, it's very important to do it in the morning, because you think so much better in the morning." I asked her about recent patterns in writing the second book that just came out. "I try to write in the morning, but I have to be very sure I get in an hour of exercise, so when it's warmer and the days are longer, it's very easy because I can walk earlier."

She was emphatic about exercising whenever and however she can. Some recent back problems have underscored the importance. "If I write first, I get so involved in it, I don't get out and walk. In theory, I'm supposed to get up and walk every half hour for my back, but you sit down and get involved, and the first thing you know, it's been an hour and a half. I try not to write in the evening. I get so into it that it interferes with falling asleep," she laughs.

A writing regime that follows exercise underscores John Ratey's observations about the boost in brain functioning, and learning in particular, especially in older folks. Based on a 2006 study at the University of Illinois, Ratey reported that "walking as few as three days a week for six months increased the volume of the prefrontal cortex in older adults. The prefrontal cortex is the home of working memory, the brain's RAM, which is crucial to decision making . . . and the CEO of most brain functions."[25] Caroline's work-exercise routine also mirrors what most of the other budding late-blooming artists reported to me.

Refocusing on her most recent undertaking, the painstaking cataloging and restoring of crumbling, yellowing letters from her father to her mother during WWI, seemed to me like a combination of museum curator and Sherlock Holmes. She demurely agreed, maybe a bit embarrassed by my comparison. But in fact, "the Bethel Museum in my home town in Connecticut, where my parents were born and I grew up, would like to have the originals." Her diligent documentation formed the basis for her second book, *Dear Hannah, Dear Pa.*

Curious about her next writing project, now that her father's World War I army service was safely ensconced in book form; Caroline is not interested in taking a break. Her mother's remarkable life, not surprisingly, is her next historical account and already underway. "She was almost a pioneer—a woman who had a career of her own and was successful at it. So, I've got her to age thirty-nine," she laughs. "I've got to get her to 107!"

No doubt the writer and historian in Caroline will tirelessly write all she recalls from the past, to preserve it and to pass down this fascinating piece of Americana while entertaining readers with her tales.

---

[25] p. 160

6   Yvette: Poet and Short Story Writer

Born into a poor, immigrant family in a Brooklyn, New York, tenement, this Depression-era baby was the youngest of five daughters. It was a very long and winding road from her humble beginnings to her cozy townhouse in the northeast which is filled with a lifetime of memories, her own art work, and her books of short stories and poems, one of which was recently published. Though I hadn't seen her in four years, we picked up exactly where we left off—talking about our family. Yvette is my aunt, my mother's youngest sister.

In truth, I always knew that she was imaginative and intensely curious about all sorts of things, but only recently did I come to learn that she was an artist, a writer, and the creative director of a cable TV station in her community. She seemed like the sort of person I wanted to interview for this book: a late-blooming artist who finally breathed life into her creative ability. And so I traveled across the country to get the rest of her story.

As if things were not bad enough when Yvette was a child, with a sickly mother and four older sisters who were teens when she was born, her father left when she was about ten years old and life got still harder. Perhaps because of her isolation, her imagination, and the absence of money for toys, she invented stories to entertain herself and later the kids in the neighborhood. Hers was a talent born of necessity; her enthralled audiences helped to sharpen her storyteller's tools.

An average student, Yvette recalled one high school teacher's words: "Someday, you're going to be a writer." She easily recalled the words as we talked, but it took forty years for her teacher's prediction to be realized. Like so many other Depression-era folks, making a living trumped staying in school. At sixteen, Yvette quit school and shortly thereafter married her high school sweetheart. The turbulent war years and the deployment of her young husband to Europe made survival her number-one goal.

At twenty-six and nine months pregnant, she graduated from night high school. "I was now a straight-A student; I felt good about myself for the first time," she recalled with a flush of pride. At thirty and the mother of two young children, she enrolled in a community college, and to her amazement: "I got an A in college!"

Intoxicated by her own achievement, she discovered a competitive part of herself who wanted more. Divorced, working, and raising three children, she managed to pursue further education during her forties and fifties, finishing a bachelor's degree in psychology with honors and a master's degree in counseling.

As Yvette told her story, I was in awe of her perseverance and tenacity, but I also understood that early hardship can make a person quite hardy. During all the years of striving, achieving, raising a family, and managing daily life, the creativity of this childhood storyteller laid dormant. The stories needed another decade to incubate.

Yvette's early talent surfaced again in her mid fifties when she began to write short stories. When I asked how she started and why, Yvette searched into her memory and sounded surprised when she recalled, "I went to visit my sister in Florida. I took an Amtrak train, and I didn't know what I was going to do for twenty-eight hours, so I took a notebook with me. When I was in Florida, a couple visited my sister. The woman had just lost her sister, and the husband couldn't stop talking about the sister. He went on and on about how wonderful she was, how beautiful she was, and I was a little shocked. He sounded like he was in love with her.

"It started a kernel of interest in their story, so on the way back home, I took out that notebook and started to write. It turned out to have eight-hundred and fifty pages!" Noticing my amazement, she clarified, "Not all on the train. I was writing like crazy, and when I got back home, I continued writing this novel. Of course, it was an exhausting experience, but I couldn't seem to end it. It just went on and on and on. So I thought, 'The next time, I'm going to write a short story. This is too much of a commitment.'" I'm not sure she intended to be humorous, but that's just her personality, and I found her short stories to be funny with just a twist of sarcasm.

Retracing her steps as a newborn writer and her marathon first attempt, Yvette mused, "I became very involved with the characters, and I think I've always been pretty imaginative. As a child, I always made up these situations and created the scenarios to act out with the kids in the neighborhood."

Still trying to understand what got stirred up inside of her that energized her to pursue the novel so relentlessly, I asked, "What did the writing do for you?" "It gave me a fantasy life, an outlet for something creative," she replied. She seemed pleased with her newfound ability. It was reassuring—maybe she was smart after all. Maybe her high school teacher was right about her.

She recalled that while working for Consolidated Edison, the giant utility in New York City, "they were having a contest for writing a jingle, so now after I had written a whole novel I wasn't worried about writing a jingle so I submitted every month that they had this contest." To insure impartiality, no names were used, but every month Yvette won and was rewarded with a $50 savings bond each time. I joked that she was now a professional, being paid and winning recognition in the company newsletter.

With renewed confidence she thought, "'I can write jingles.' So I started writing poetry for the company newspaper." She took some risks, which were reinforced just enough to feed her passion.

By sixty-five, her creative juices were flowing in all directions but retirement wasn't meant to be. Learning bridge at the local senior center didn't excite her, so as a lark she became a substitute teacher at a neighborhood elementary school. "One day, I drew a large tiger on the chalkboard, and the principal came in." Three days later, Yvette was offered a job as an art teacher. With no fine-arts experience, she reinvented herself. "I wondered, where the heck did this all come from? I didn't know I could do this. I worked there until I was seventy-six. An art teacher out of nowhere!"

Yvette was on a roll. More confident than ever, she craved time and space, left teaching behind, and moved to a retirement community where her short-story writing blossomed and a couple of her books were published.

As it is with so many older adults, daily life in the twenties, thirties, forties, and even fifties gets in the way of the child-like curiosity that finally bubbles up when the should-do demands lessen. With Yvette summing up her life in an hour, it is amazing to see how her creative trajectory skyrocketed when her path was unimpeded.

Learning these facts about a family member whom I thought I knew quite well left me stunned. I had no idea about this woman's tenacity, drive, and later-in-life talent. Sensing my surprise she was quick to add, "It was a long road. It wasn't easy. Self discovery came hard."

Trying to better understand and possibly even predict someone's artistic temperament, which can lie dormant for so many years but blossom when nourished later in life, I looked around for psychological theories that might be useful. One such idea is an offshoot of a concept suggested by Carl Jung, the neurologist who was a colleague of Sigmund Freud until he branched out to form his own school of psychoanalysis.

The concept known as the shadow is the unconscious and unrealizable part of oneself that finds expression in indirect ways. Followers of Jung may find this extrapolation a bit farfetched and even a misunderstanding of Jung, but it helps explain what I saw in Yvette's life. If we can assume that she was always creative, imaginative, and artistic, but that her early life could not provide the outlets for expressing these attributes, it would make sense that her shadow, her creative self, might be channeled some other way.

Here are some possible channels. Her firstborn child became an artist. Not just a painter, but also a champion for the rights of street artists in New York City. He defends their interests, articulates their concerns, and represents them in court proceedings. Her second son has always played the guitar but also composes and writes lyrics. How Yvette may have infused their choices with her own interests is not obvious, but it really is a common scenario observed by those of us who study people.

Looking into her distant past, it is probably not an accident that when World War II ended, Yvette's husband worked as a commercial artist by day and a painter after dark. She certainly didn't influence his talent or occupation directly, but she chose him for a life partner possibly sensing the artistry that he could—but she could not—express at that time.

Jung's shadow concept may be a stretch to explain Yvette's marriage, but other theories explore how people choose partners to complete themselves or to live through another's experience vicariously when their own path is blocked or simply not available. Here is another fact: Yvette's second husband of thirty-five years was a musician, and served as a member of the Army Special Services during World War II entertaining troops in Europe. He continued to play the saxophone professionally until he died, and in his later years was also a fine artist who created intricate designs resembling mandalas, the geometric art forms associated with Buddhist and Hindu traditions.

Yvette's current boyfriend is not an artist, writer, or musician, but in conversation with him recently, he was wondering what it would be like to learn the violin—a long time passion but played only on CDs. He is eighty-five, a bit unbalanced as he walks, but strong enough to carry a violin case, hold a bow and press on a string. He was encouraged by my recent cello exploration.

Returning from fancy speculation to our interview, I asked Yvette for some words of wisdom for others who are nearing retirement age and wondering how to live their later years. With barely a pause she responded, "Don't be afraid to change lanes. You haven't even scratched the surface. We all have such untapped potential that we don't know about, and maybe we go through life without discovering it if we haven't experimented and journeyed away from the usual." She confirmed other interviewees' experiences. The Vintage Years give you time and permission to explore life in new ways and to complete the picture, because time's running out.

Knowing about Yvette's significant physical problems during the past five years, I asked how her artistic endeavors affect or are affected by health issues. "I think that my need to be creative is a very good distraction from the unfortunate reality of having health issues. I think that every time I try something new, every time I try to branch out with another skill or another challenge, I think it keeps my brain young, as young as it can be at this point." Research on body-brain functioning mirrors her perception. Being immersed in a pleasurable activity creates a time-out from pain and worry.

Cueing her about any possible interest in leaving a legacy through her writing and art, which are tangible and can be handed down to the next few generations, she said, "I don't think about that. It's more the process I enjoy, the satisfaction. Without being conscious of it, I wanted to attain self-actualization. I didn't give it a name, but that's what I wanted."

In summing up her life to this point, she is doing that which gives her meaning and pleasure, living her life on her own terms, and enjoying the process of learning and discovery. I'd call that self-actualization!

7 Bette: Writer and Sketch Artist

I was told in advance that I would love Bette and that her life was extraordinary. Both are true. She lives in a retirement community in a small, cramped apartment that, at the moment, she shares with her middle-aged daughter and regal cat, Marbles, so named for the pattern of his fur coat. The two rooms were so stuffed with papers, books, sundries, and furniture that it took some effort to navigate around things in getting to my seat on the folded futon. I perched my tape recorder on the edge of a storage box that held a tray, papers, and knickknacks.

At eighty-two, Bette is the picture of health: petite, slim, beaming through a virtually line-free face, dressed in jeans and sandals. The first glimpse does not even begin to tell her story, as her life has been anything but privileged and smooth. In fact, it has only been during the past sixteen years that her art has flourished. Not by accident, her writing and sketching coincides with the years she has been living at Sunny View, the longest stretch in her life with consistent housing. Thanks to her Social Security and SSI check, she is able to live here without the worry of being dispossessed. As time and greater peace have allowed, she writes copiously and sketches mostly cartoon-like animals.

Bette sat across from me and candidly unfolded her life almost without stopping to breathe. Any of her stories could have been a book in itself. She preferred to start her tale at the beginning, and so will I in telling it.

Born to two schoolteachers in a small college town in Minnesota, Bette began to draw at a young age but without encouragement from her family. Rather, it was the opposite.

Both parents discouraged what she called creativity and took a very strong negative stance about starving artists. It struck me as odd, since her father was a piano teacher. Unlike Mozart, whose father taught him, inspired him, or at least guided him and managed his early music life, Bette's father was opposed to her pursuing any formal training as an artist or musician. This is particularly ironic, because she could play the piano by the age of three. He pushed her toward the safety of becoming a teacher, which she rebelled against from the beginning.

Unlike her conventional Minnesota family, Bette wasn't content to stay put and moved wherever work took her after college, "from Minneapolis to Boston, where I was a singer and guitarist." As if anticipating my next question, she pulled out a publicity photo of herself wearing white boots and supporting a guitar on her lap, looking like a country-western singer from the 70s, big hair and all. "I got work because I wasn't on drugs, didn't smoke, and didn't drink," she said, suggesting that her reliability increased her value in spite of her significant health problems, including childhood Type 1 diabetes. "I have an insulin pump which has kept me alive all these years," she said as she enumerated additional medical challenges. Playing in various hotels in Boston and Martha's Vineyard kept her busy for a couple of years. Though she finally felt secure in her music profession, "it was cut short when I developed tendonitis in both elbows, which you use while playing the guitar," she mimicked strumming an imaginary guitar in the air, "and my diabetes became very difficult to control."

The condo, which she bought while recuperating and hoping to return to her music career, ultimately went into foreclosure when her health took a further nosedive. "The sheriff came one day and put me out, which was pretty terrifying." She decided to go back home when, "The doctors told me I had a year to live. I was having up to eight insulin reactions a day." The low blood sugar seriously impacted her ability to think, and she was no longer able to work as a singer.

As you might expect, going back to Minnesota didn't work out, and when her health improved enough for her to be mobile, Bette went back to Boston. Unable to resume her career and needing to support herself, she worked at odd jobs—like assistant housemaster in a Harvard dormitory—"where at a party I met a young fella who played the cello. His name was Yo Yo Ma. He would come in every Sunday and play for us." She beamed and swayed as she vividly recalled the pleasure of the music. Later, she worked as a caretaker and companion to a string of older wealthy matrons. Many of these positions were temporary. "I would work six months and then move on." These gigs were interesting and gave Bette a glimpse into the lifestyles of the ultra-wealthy.

One such position brought her to California, then terminated abruptly. Her life continued to focus on day-to-day survival. She agreed with my observation that she could cope with just about anything, but surviving isn't enough to satisfy the needs of the heart and soul. Fortunately, at sixty-six, she found her current subsidized apartment and finally she "could do the things I wanted to do—the artwork, the writing."

Though feeling blessed these last sixteen years, she's had numerous physical problems: breaks in both shoulders and legs plus four vertebrae, for example, as a result of a seizure-like insulin reaction. "I began to write in my late sixties, and then I began to draw. I had a lot of stories to tell, and I wanted to get them down." Her life was so serious until that point that she "needed to write something a little more fanciful."

She continued, "Loving cats and Sherlock Holmes, I put the two together and wrote a story about 'Catlock,' a cat who lived with Sherlock Holmes—a curious cat who does some investigating." Displaying my own curiosity I asked what writing did for her; she lit up and nearly shouted, "It brought me tremendous joy," at which point she whipped out a series of sketched cartoon cats, more caricatures than exact representations and very humorous, one with a broad smile on his face. We both laughed at the sight of them.

"I'm doing quite well," she went on. "I know which way I'm going and what I want to accomplish, if God willing I live long enough. *Catlock*, the book, is finished, with just a few chapters left to revise." She continues to write freehand, goes to her retirement complex's writing group every two weeks, and works this around daily insulin tests to keep her blood sugar stable.

As if anticipating my final question she volunteered, "It doesn't matter what you choose to do, but do it, just do it. Don't let other things take precedence," Bette preaches to the choir. "It's very easy to turn the TV on and watch other people's lives. Use TV to feed your creativity." This is Bette's advice to those approaching the Vintage Years. Looking forward, with a chuckle in her voice, she wonders about a sequel to *Catlock* and what she'll pen after that.

8 Wisdom: Enhancing the Arts

It's not the years in your life that count. It's the life in your years.
—Abraham Lincoln

A lifetime accumulation of knowledge and experience, with the added bonus of a calmer more focused brain, drives the process that leads to wisdom. Wisdom is a fitting compensation for aging.

Henry, the wood sculptor you met in Part II, personifies wisdom. At ninety-six, he has weathered just about every storm that life has thrown at him. His decades of life experience inform his current decision making without much effort. The patterning that takes place in the prefrontal lobe of his brain's cerebral cortex occurs mostly without his awareness and in a shorthand that doesn't require consciously analyzing all the data. Little effort is needed here.

While Henry's memory for the specifics of what happened in his distant past is quite good, the same can be said for most Vintage-Years folks. What happened long ago remains as clear as glass. Henry also has the good fortune of being able to remember what happened in the near past, even last week and yesterday!

He retrieves the words he wishes on command—something more difficult for many of us in the Vintage Years.

But even if he couldn't remember a name, or misplaced his keys, or couldn't recall what he ate for dinner or saw at the movies, he would still have the benefit of the compensating processes and cognitive reserve available later in life. He could still explain his meaning and find other words, since older adults process tasks across broader regions of the brain. According to Goldberg, author of *The Wisdom Paradox*, "The repertoire of patterns grows with age. So aging is the price we must pay for accumulating wisdom patterns".[26]

Henry is an extraordinary man by any account, and at his advanced age very different from the man of his youth—in positive ways, according to him. In spite of some mobility problems, for which he uses a walker, he shows patience and tolerance for himself. He accepts and appreciates what he can do and shows little of the frustration and irritation you might expect to see in a younger person striving to be better, to do more, or to accomplish something quickly.

As he looks back over nearly a century, he does so with an expanded perspective. He views his life at a glance and feels content to have the busyness of an achieving life behind him. While he speaks of the past, he prefers the present where he passionately pursues his arts and where time unfolds on a daily basis without pressure. His Vintage Years, once filled with hours of woodcarving, are now filled with a less physically demanding hobby in his nineties: building complex, three-dimensional dioramas out of paper. Rather than feeling bitter at having to give

---

[26] p.154

up his satisfying hobby, he saw the change as an exciting segue to a new art. His expanded perception both enhances and benefits from his wisdom, informed by nearly a century of life expe-experience.

Though his secondary career as an artist didn't begin until he was sixty-eight, Henry summed up his past without a pause, as if his life was a painting in full view. "We made our own toys back then. When I was seven years old, I made my first carving: an elephant out of a cake of white ivory soap. It's yellow now. I still have it if you want to see it. I'll show it to you." He laughed at the memory and the aging elephant, and without missing a beat, fast-forwarded to the creative years that came much later. Seamlessly traversing a lifetime, he brought us back to the present and the paper constructions, his current passion. They are novel, complex, and evolve day-to-day as he resolves whatever technical problems he encounters—just the right ingredients to keep his aging brain buzzing along optimally.

Wisdom and the Brain

Like Henry, everything we've done with our brains up to this point is still paying off. Simply living our lives, making daily decisions, and learning from the outcomes can, with a little help, lead us to a vibrant senior life. Our brain's capacity is limitless, unlike our computers. The more we use our brains for new and engaging reasons, the more robust they become and the greater protection they provide against decay.

But the brain is more than a storehouse crammed with data. It's a complex organ that is informed by your emotions, judgments, hormones, and interpersonal relationships. It keeps evolving, and it responds positively to good care and good "food." It's never too late to pump up your brain-fitness routine to optimally strengthen your cognitive sharpness, and you can do so until your last day on earth. So even if you haven't challenged yourself until a recent health scare or a bout of senior-forgetting moments, your brain is forgiving and will work with you on any new strengthening regimen. You can begin a process of further developing your brain directly through learning and practicing something complex and stimulating anytime you wish. Or you can challenge your body physically, to whatever extent possible, and your brain will continue to develop from widespread neuronal activation.

The wisdom that accompanies our senior years also benefits from the emotional steadiness that often characterizes this stage of life. The brain signals the production of estrogen and testosterone, the gender-specific hormones, and knows to decrease production around the same time that fertility is no longer necessary in women and competitiveness and physical prowess slows in men. This is partly why postmenopausal women and men of about the same age feel calmer, less driven.

The decrease and eventual leveling out of estrogen, progesterone, and testosterone lead to better judgments and less emotionally-driven decisions in both men and women. Louis Cozolino echoes this in his book about the healthy aging brain. He points to the biological factors that underpin wisdom and the "slower processing and advanced neural integration leading to more thoughtful deliberation".[27] This is the trade off: slower processing but greater emotional integration, self-awareness and

_____

[27] p.128

perspective. Couple this with a lifetime of experience and you have a cornerstone for building wisdom.

Based on a huge number of experiences, the aging brain doesn't need to approach each situation as if it were novel. Over a lifetime, the frontal cortex automated many processes through pattern formation. It uses a shorthand system to determine if something is familiar or not, and if it is, it searches within its archives for a way to handle or resolve it behaviorally. This patterning is done with little or no awareness on our part.

We are decidedly at an advantage over younger folks, as our repertoire of events is so much larger based at least on a longer timeline. What is new to the younger brain is often second nature to an older brain. Another way to say this is that an older person can run through their repertoire of experiences very rapidly, like a computer doing a search, while a younger person has fewer bits of data on which to build a problem's solution.

With the frontal cortex humming along, due to the benefit of a long life rich in problem solving, there is a shift to the parietal region of the brain, found near the top of the head above the ears. This is where the senses and conscious thought are integrated and is the "executive region of inner experience just as the frontal lobes are an executive region for behavior,"[28] according to Cozolino. What this means is that there is an increased shift to inner experience and self-awareness because attention to the outside world can be handled more automatically. The bonus is enhanced creativity, perfect for taking up the arts.

Tapping a vast store of memories, having less of a need to handle every new situation from scratch, and possessing greater

---

[28] p.179

emotional resilience and increased self-knowledge gives the aging but new artist a capacity for approaching and managing creative pursuits in ways not possible before this point in life. Add to this mix fewer distractions from the outside world and the ability to focus due to slower cognitive processing speed, and you have the increased likelihood of *flow* that we talked about in Chapter 4, the ability to be so absorbed that time and the outside world tend to disappear. Henry is a poster boy for the wise old man: knowing, emotionally centered, and curious.

Wisdom and Evolutionary Psychology

Wisdom is the product of a long and interesting life, cumulative decision-making, and stored patterns to facilitate new learning. That it first buds in the Vintage Years helps explain the value of elders in human history. The relatively new field of evolutionary psychology suggests that the cognitive programs of the human brain are really adaptations. They exist because they produced behavior in our ancestors that enabled them to survive and reproduce. But what exactly is the survival value of wisdom?

In the very distant past, and to some extent even in the present, the oldest amongst us were not able to run fast and they didn't have excellent vision, the physical agility to hunt, or the endurance to tolerate exhausting labor day after day. But elders contributed something less tangible to communal well-being still worthy of support. They were the repositories of knowledge, the "hard drives" of that era.

In the history of the human species, elders provided a link between past and present. They provided a big-picture perspective, dispassionate judgment, and level-headedness often lacking in the young. What a useful commodity in fighting wars, anticipating future events, and in general making sense out of life!

Whether you refer to the aging member of the clan as wise one, shaman, medicine person, or sage, the idea is the same. The wise older brain can chronicle and express a collection of ideas to multiple generations. Also, at this point in life, art has richness, ripeness, and depth not possible before, enhanced by aging like fine wine and the best cheese.

Wisdom and Aging Artists from the Past

Purportedly, Michelangelo said during the last years of his life, "I'm still learning." At seventy-four, he was appointed architect for Saint Peter's Basilica and designed its famous dome. It is true that he was a creative genius who, in his early twenties, painted twelve thousand square feet of the Sistine Chapel ceiling. Certainly there are others whose artistry blossomed early, but they are so rare that their names are household words—like Mozart.

The Vivaldis of music or Picassos of art began early and continued to produce brilliant works into their senior years. The art they created in their last years, as wonderful as the early versions were, continued to evolve and deepen. Such is the effect of wisdom on art.

In *Lastingness: The Art of Old Age,* Delbanco actually reversed his original premise that artists lose their creativity or that their talent diminishes as they age. He noted that a writer at sixty, for example, couldn't have produced what he did twenty years before. The painter at seventy could not have produced that art half a century before, and "the composer in her eighties hears a different tonal register than does the forty-year-old".[29]

Delbanco said that art in the later years serves a different purpose than it initially did. For his father-in-law Bernard Greenhouse, a cellist and founding member of the renowned classical chamber music ensemble Beaux Arts Trio, "music - making in and of itself sustains him; indeed it keeps him young." The pleasures still provided by playing cello at ninety-four "outweighed the sorrow of lessened effect".[30]

The goals of the older artists are different from their youthful selves. Referring to artists as they age, Delbanco suggests, "The making of the thing itself displaces its reception; reviews and sales and standing ovations come to matter less".[31] The private or inner world of the artist matters more, and satisfaction is internal, experienced for its own sake. This is consistent with all the research which shows that brain changes that affect an older person's goals and motivation to be much more intrinsic and much less comparative and competitive.

"If time is the great teacher," says Delbanco, "a senior artist ought to have earned wisdom to depart. She or he may grow more venturesome, less trammeled by propriety...once there seems less to lose."[32] And so it is for the budding, late-blooming artists you've encountered in this book, armed with wisdom and

---

[29] p. 198

[30] p. 215

[31] p. 217

[32] p. 205

little worry about what others think of their art; their ripeness explodes with passion.

Ralph Vaughn Williams, the preeminent British composer of the 20th century, composed his ninth and final symphony when he was eighty-six years old. While it's true that he was musical from the time he was a young child, he went on to do some of his finest work in his last two symphonies when he was past eighty-two.

If in fact the brain's capacity diminishes, then one would hardly expect such creativity and artistry in someone in their eighth decade, cut short only by his death a few months after the ninth symphony was complete. What very likely contributed to the brilliance and majesty of his last two symphonies was a lifetime of experience, coupled with self-knowledge and knowledge of the world, making his music reflect all of who he had fully become.

In spite of his family wealth and lineage, Vaughn Williams volunteered to be an infantry soldier in WWI where he saw unspeakable horrors and lost six close friends. Further intensifying his emotional experiences, his wife of fifty years suffered with chronic pain and was wheelchair bound for nine-tenths of their marriage. In photographs depicting their relationship, he is standing over her, lovingly attending to her. But the demand of never being able to be away from her side seems to have exacted a toll. The psychological pain he experienced, or so his biographers say, created a certain emotional awareness that he infused into his music. Researchers refer to this quality as wisdom, the accumulation of knowledge of self and the outside world that becomes integrated later in life.

Pablo Picasso also showed promise as a young child and continued to evolve as an artist whose influence spanned almost the entire twentieth century until his death at ninety-two. His paintings were done over a series of stages informed by what he saw in his early years in the outside world, like poverty in Spain, circus life, war, and his trip to Africa which inspired his sculptures that heralded the first phase of cubism.

In a recent showing of Picasso's collective works in San Francisco, on loan from the Louvre while the museum was undergoing revamping, I was struck by the tremendous differences in style between the young and the old Picasso. While I am not a visual artist and have little sophistication in understanding the evolution of a painter, I could see how volatile moods, sad emotion, and the loss of various mistresses influenced his earlier phases like the Blue Period. The agony he felt about the 1937 bombing of the Spanish town of Guernica led to his landmark painting titled *Guernica*, which was a condemnation of war that he painted when he was fifty-six.

Toward the end of his life when his brain, influenced by normal aging, turned his attention toward the inner world and his more introspective side, his creations leaned toward fantasy and comic invention. He continued to explore and express new aspects of his personal vision until he died. A sense of peacefulness, to which the aging brain contributes, seems to have had a calming effect on the elderly Picasso. Only days before he died, he is said to have told a friend, "Death holds no fear for me. It has a kind of beauty. What I am afraid of is falling ill and not being able to work. That's lost time."[33]

---

[33] *TIME Magazine*; April 23, 1973

Wisdom is interwoven with the search for and expression of what is personally meaningful, and Picasso in his final days felt the urgency to complete the projects that were to be his ultimate contribution to the world and his unique legacy. This is wisdom at work.

Wisdom, Exercise, and the Brain: Creating Synergy

"If you have a better, stronger, more connected brain going over the hill, it will surely be more resilient and resist neuronal breakdown that much longer,"[34] says John Ratey, M.D., an expert on the relationship between physical exercise and the brain. Even with, and maybe especially with, an older population, he provides scientific evidence of exercise's benefits, like increased neural activity caused by the increased blood volume produced by physical exercise.

Recognizing the limitations associated with aging, Dr. Ratey is not proposing mountain climbing or wind surfing, although some eighty-year-olds are perfectly capable of engaging in these hobbies. He says, "Any motor skill more complicated than walking has to be learned and thus it challenges the brain".[35] So, the bar is set rather low and attainable for most of us.

Ratey reports on a landmark research study completed in 2006 at the University of Illinois that confirmed through MRI scans that "walking as few as three days a week for six months increased the volume of the prefrontal cortex in older adults".[36]

---

[34] p. 223

[35] p. 56

[36] p. 160

Keep in mind that the prefrontal cortex is the most newly evolved part of the brain. This gray matter imbues us with the quintessential human capacity for understanding, planning, and judging. Our working memory resides here as well, and working memory is subject to deterioration as we age. For example, recalling someone's name, or a movie title, or even what you ate for dinner last night, is not the sturdiest ability of the aging brain.

Dr. Ratey is an exemplar of the well-exercised brain. At sixty, his exercise routine is as regular a part of his life as brushing teeth before bed at night. While we'll never know how much his daily workout contributes to the sharpness and productivity that led to his writing eight books and maintaining a professorship at Harvard Medical School, he clearly practices what he preaches.

Since it works for him, I thought I would share his routine with you: "I got into the habit of doing weights plus crunches and balance exercises two times a week, three times when I'm really focused. The other days I do forty minutes on the elliptical trainer, or on the treadmill when I want to add in some intervals".[37] Recently, he added a few sprints while on the treadmill which paid off with a bit of weight loss around his middle by stimulating human growth hormones, or HGH, that increase muscle mass and energy in natural ways.

If reading this makes you laugh a little guiltily as you recognize the disparity between Ratey's physical self-challenges and your own, take a breath and let me break this down another way. Keep in mind that your goal is not to compete in the World Olympics but to stimulate your aging brain through exercise,

[37] p. 266

just enough to keep neuronal and hormonal production at stimulating levels.

Why is this important? When you exercise, especially shortly before doing a learning activity, the synergy between exercise, the brain being stimulated, and wisdom is at its optimal level. You met Caroline in Part II. Exercising before writing is her habit. She began writing memoirs at eighty. At ninety, she writes daily after taking a long walk in the county park adjacent to her active-senior complex.

Facilitated by exercise, the patterns stored in your brain over decades of learning and a vast number of experiences are open to take in new information that will be incorporated into the existing patterns. "Pattern-recognition capacity comprises a very important element of wisdom,"[38] according to Goldberg, author of the *Wisdom Paradox*. He suggests that the patterns that facilitate problem solving in the older brain are based on generic memories that, unlike the content of yesterday's experience, accumulate with age and are unlikely to deteriorate.

The energy produced by exercising prior to problem solving or learning something new, in your art for example, will keep you alert and focused. Think of it as having a double espresso before writing a poem, practicing a new piece of music, or finishing the oil painting that needs just one more touch.

Dr. Ratey's daily physicality may seem daunting, but the principles are easy to modify. Any trainer will tell you that you need three components to your workout for maximal benefit: weight training for muscle fitness and bone density; cardiovascular exercise through fast walking, jogging, treadmill, or

---

[38] p.149

elliptical trainer; and flexibility gained through yoga or other kinds of stretching. Even a few minutes of each spread over the course of a week in some kind of daily pursuit has a tremendous cumulative effect, not just on the body but on the brain as well.

Finally, if this argument isn't persuasive enough, consider that in evolutionary terms, our bodies and brains were programmed for a human species when it was in its evolutionary infancy. "Our genes are coded for this activity, and our brains are meant to direct it. Take that activity away, and you're disrupting a delicate biological balance that has been fine-tuned over half a million years,"[39] says Ratey.

It turns out that relatively sedentary routines, consistent with twenty-first century lifestyles, don't really satisfy the brain's need for challenge and stimulation. Here is the super-simplistic bottom line: keep the wisdom growing by doing something physical every day.

Remember ninety-six year old Henry? He uses a walker but still makes time daily for arm strengthening using five-pound weights and leg lifts using his own body weight. When we met at his home, he was not content to just tell me but grabbed his blue rubber-coated weights to demonstrate his practice. Then he proceeded to do a few leg lifts just to prove his point. If you don't have Henry's mobility, adaptive techniques are definitely available from your trainer or physical therapist.

One of the best-known studies examining the role of exercise and continued learning to challenge the brain involves a sect of teaching nuns in rural Minnesota. This longitudinal study began in 1986, under the direction of epidemiologist David Snowdon of

[39] p. 248

the University of Minnesota, and continues to this day. While the original goal of the study was to understand and maybe predict the likelihood of developing Alzheimer's disease by studying a group of similar individuals over time, there were some unexpected and fascinating findings.

Many of the nuns live well into their nineties and beyond, which is not surprising in a convent environment where social, spiritual, and economic support combines with low stress. The lifestyle within the convent includes daily exercise. I can testify, having seen a video of several nuns with an average age of ninety-five exercising, that the equipment they use includes weights and machines that can be found in any fitness club.

I watched Sister Esther, interviewed at age 102, cycling on a recumbent elliptical trainer while she talked breathlessly about her age and the study in which she agreed to participate. She arranged to leave her brain to science so that after her death it can be determined whether, in spite of her articulateness and vigorous physical routine, she had the markers for Alzheimer's disease.

What is surprising, according to Dr. Snowdon, is that while half of the sisters have normal brains when they die, "a significant number of them have full blown Alzheimer's disease in the brain yet are acting normally."[40] Interestingly, they don't seem to manifest the memory loss and physical failings that you might expect to see with Alzheimer's disease.

The explanation seems to rest with the level of mental and physical activity that nuns like Sister Esther engage in on a daily basis even in their old age. Sister Jane Frances is ninety-five and

---

[40] see video: http://sciencehack.com/videos/view/nw2lafKIEio).

was assembling a one-thousand-piece puzzle as she spoke to the interviewer. "They tell me that if you work puzzles, you can keep your mind active, so I puzzle."[41] Then there was 103-year-old Sister Mathia who knits to stay focused. In the video, she was working four needles in a complex pattern as she talked about the need to have an active mind and to keep thinking.

By having as active a mind as possible, combined with physical exercise to whatever extent possible, an older brain can indeed compensate for some damage and deterioration. Dr. Snowdon refers to this ability as cognitive reserve, the enhanced ability to recruit alternate brain networks as needed. This is an example of very positive compensation.

While the sisters did not talk explicitly about the arts, I would not be at all surprised if there were some water colorists, flutists, and authors in their midst. Whether this is true is not as important as the fact that engaging in an art form provides the complexity necessary to keep your brain in tip-top shape. Like the nuns, however, you need to practice on a regular basis for your remaining years to derive the cognitive benefits just described.

Malcolm Gladwell, the best-selling author well known for his keen and fascinating observations of human nature, captured the difference between young and late-blooming artists in his 2008 short story, "What the Dog Saw." In describing Cezanne's and Mark Twain's trial-and-error style, which is characteristic of late bloomers, he points out that their kind of creativity "takes a long

---

[41] Ibid.

time to come to fruition".[42] It doesn't have the precocity that we usually think about with brilliant artists, like Wolfgang Mozart, who were stars early on.

Referring to Cezanne's inability to draw as a young man, Gladwell quips, "Let's just be thankful that Cezanne didn't have a guidance counselor in high school who looked at his primitive sketches and told him to try accounting".[43] Such was actually the plight of a number of the late-blooming artists you met in Part II, who postponed or abandoned any thoughts of their artistry as kids or young adults because their abilities weren't manifest back then or they didn't have a benefactor to support their lifestyle while they did their art.

Wisdom comes later in life and requires many decades of experience and acquired knowledge, coupled with mature judgment that informs the artist and the art. This is what creates the late-blooming artist whose talent could not possibly have blossomed earlier. The continuous learning of a wise elder is the ultimate stimulant for the brain.

Sealing the Wisdom: Summing-Up and Encore

Dr. Gene Cohen, whose life-stage taxonomy we looked at in the chapter 4, identified the last phases of development as "summing-up and encore." These comprise the years from about seventy until the end of life. He suggests that individuals at this point are fully aware of the clock running out and have the urgent "desire to find larger meaning in the story of their lives

---

[42] p. 303

[43] p. 305

through a process of reviewing, summarizing, and giving back".[44]

According to Cohen, this is perfect timing because "the use of both sides of the brain allows for an optimal expression of the full range of factual and emotional elements in a person's life story ".[45] By utilizing the right and left hippocampi in recalling memories, the thinking brain (neocortical) links with the feeling brain (limbic system). At long last, the feeling and thinking parts of the brain are working across both hemispheres, reaching a sort of crescendo, a peak time for consolidating a lifetime and possibly immortalizing one's contribution to the world in writing, song, or visual imagery. Combine this with more vivid emotionality and the desire to give back in the form of storytelling and memoirs—these are the ingredients that define wisdom.

In Cohen's comprehensive and well-designed study of seventy and eighty–year-olds enrolled in visual, music, and writing arts programs, conducted in conjunction with the National Endowment for the Arts, he noted a large number of individuals were writing memoirs or engaged in other types of creative life reviews. Even for the oldest subjects in Cohen's study, "the ever-evolving Inner Push for growth and development has a positive impact".[46]

The hypothesis in his landmark research was, "The people who participated in the multifaceted arts programs would show less decline than the control group who did not participate in

---

[44] *The Mature Mind*, p. 75

[45] p. 76

[46] p. 85

those programs".[47] After one year, the preliminary results were very positive for the participants compared to the control group. The group that participated in the arts programs:

- had better health after one year
- had fewer doctor visits
- used fewer medications
- felt less depressed
- were less lonely
- had higher morale
- were more socially active

The wise elder artists we got to know in Part II presented a rich variety of life experiences, personalities, and temperaments, very different from one another in many ways, but all demonstrating passion in expressing their arts. I can't help but feel that the quality of their lives is linked to their daily pursuits. Exercising both mind and body may also account for their general good health, mirroring the findings of Cohen's study. Being better able to use both sides of the brain, especially the hippocampi, allows elders to draw upon vast life experiences and add richness to the task of memory recall, enhancing their overall sense of wonder and awe of life.

The next chapter will help you begin the process that leads to the artist's life.

[47] p. 178

9 Making it Happen

It is never too late to be what we might have been.
—George Eliot

Time is such a paradox. A backward glance over a lifetime can feel like the blink of an eye even though it's a lengthy journey from childhood to the Vintage Years. On a day-to-day basis, time seems endless since the perspective is so narrow. But broaden out the scope, and you can capture decades-long pictures in a single glance. As we get older, this becomes easier and easier to do. Pick a decade in your own life and your memory will take you back there instantly.

Remember your childhood. Were you the one who painstakingly braided a lanyard in summer camp, or drummed on pots with wooden mixing spoons on the kitchen floor, or invented stories to fascinate your little friends? Experiences like these are never forgotten and sometimes come to mind faster than the title of the movie you saw last night. Such is the nature of memory in later life.

Can you recall the hours and days of unselfconscious play and artistic exploration that ultimately gave way to the structure of school and its demands? Art projects suddenly had to be just so—no coloring outside of the lines. Self-expression yielded to performance, which led to judgments—yours and others. For many of us, this spelled the end, or at least dormancy, of artistic expression.

Next came adulthood and the long hiatus from arts-for-fun: years of living life, growing, achieving, amassing, and finally coming up for air at fifty-five or sixty only to discover a whole new chapter ready to unfold. If this is where you find yourself, the path to the future depends on many disparate factors, including your personality, temperament, interests, financial situation, and available time, just to name a few considerations. All of these factors affect not just retirement planning but shape all the years still to come.

Retirement: Rule In or Rule Out

Age sixty-five doesn't automatically signal retirement in the twenty-first century, but it can serve to prompt internal dialogue, at least about the pros and cons. The first wave of the baby-boomer generation has already faced and crossed the threshold into the Vintage Years and Medicare. Surviving the plethora of choices that Medicare requires may be more difficult than anything that follows!

Thinking through the factors that will guide your retirement decision-making is critical, and fortunately there are abundant books and web sites to help. I've included a few titles that might prove helpful below. But in this book, the primary emphasis is on ways to go about pursuing the arts with determination and passion, whether or not you retire. Retirement isn't necessarily a prerequisite for taking up an art form. If you do retire, however, the options for practice are greatly expanded.

If the retirement decision is a done deal for you, the next section may seem more like a review; you may choose to skip it altogether. Recalling the stories of those I interviewed, as well as current professional thinking on this subject, the decision tree that follows will help those of you who are undecided to identify some factors to consider. Remember, retirement decisions are complex and multi-faceted, so you will benefit from exploring internal as well as external factors.

Decision Tree 1

A decision tree makes the process of retirement decision-making more manageable by providing a visual tool. Remember the old adage: a picture is worth a thousand words. Having said that, a few words about retirement sets the stage.

The word *retirement* itself can evoke thoughts and feelings of a shift from active to passive, from the sense of further contributing to the world to the image of riding down the proverbial hill. Attitudes, feelings, and perceptions are at least as important as any facts under consideration. Your emotional take determines whether you continue to work, embrace letting go of your work or profession, or go reluctantly and even fearfully into the next phase of life. Your personal history also colors your decision-making process.

The wisdom that fully blossoms in the later years insures well-informed choices based on years of making judgments about how to live life—what works for you and what doesn't. Decisions made during the Vintage Years will be your most robust yet, informed by accumulated self-knowledge, a sense of the world around you, and of course wisdom, which we focused on in the last chapter.

The first decision tree on the following page begins the process of exploring which way to go. Trace the steps you've already taken and see where you might place yourself today. If you find that your own process goes beyond this point, then skip to Decision Tree 2 later in this chapter.

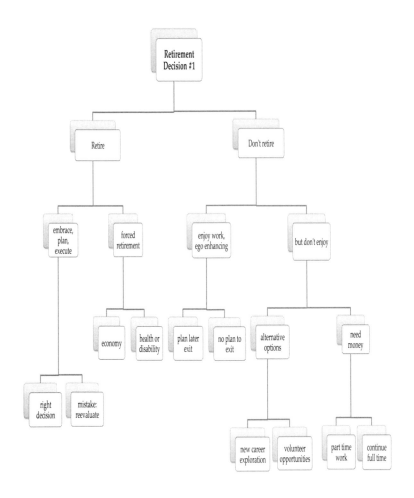

The factors detailed on the previous page may be a lot to take in all at once, but we'll analyze them sequentially and logically. They are forced choices to get you started, but retirement decisions aren't necessarily binary: retire or don't retire. A third position might be, "I don't know what to do."

To my surprise, few people in my study were undecided at sixty. Most eagerly waited for a time when they could free themselves from the shackles of work responsibilities. Clearly, mine is a biased sample, as large numbers of people never leave the work force entirely, because they don't want to or find it financially unrealistic. In truth, it's difficult to generalize from a small sample which, while equally divided between men and women and encompassing ages fifty-five to ninety-six, didn't represent a cross section of people from all socio-economic groups and ethnicities. Most of the budding late-blooming artists in my study didn't have a plan for post-retirement. Some were comfortable with this awareness and some were not.

The Influence of Personal Style

Remember Harold? He is the stained-glass artist in my study who moved to an active-senior community at sixty-five without a plan or even a worry about how to spend time only to find that fix-it projects at home were not enough to sustain his interest or pleasure. On the other hand, Gene was not comfortable thinking about retiring without a clear plan for spending his time. In fact, his retirement was tied to his subsequent strategy. His personal style required a certain next step that was, in some ways, an extension of his orderly life and career trajectory. It helped that he envisioned the life of a painter, clearly recalling his cousin's basement studio in Brooklyn and a very powerful olfactory memory—the smell of paint.

The same was true for Dan, who retired from an ophthalmology practice to enroll in a four-year art school. He began the life of an undergraduate student only a week after saying goodbye to thirty years of medical practice. But he approached this decision the way he lived life, in an orderly and systematic way—well thought out and planned prior to retirement, to be executed the moment he made his exit from work.

Frankly, the absence of much ambivalence about what to do with one's life after sixty was a surprising finding. I would have expected more internal struggle in making that decision. Maybe my surprise was colored by my decades of psychology practice helping countless decision makers become unstuck or resolve their ambivalence.

In general, those who were interviewed for this book were psychologically stable and healthy with the typical struggles of daily life that we all encounter. Clinical psychologists tend to study pathology, disease, and that which is psychologically unhealthy or in need of repair. I need to remind myself that most people ride the waves of life—the disappointments, losses, and even traumatic experiences—quite successfully. The folks I interviewed seemed resourceful, positive, and adaptive. I assume this is true for most of the readers of this book.

The professionals among the participants I interviewed—medical doctors, lawyers, and accountants, to name a few—didn't cling to the identity provided by their licenses any more than the butchers and sales people. The men who identified very closely with their work did not seem to have more difficulty walking away from jobs than did the women in my study. This surprised me. Moving on didn't seem to strip anyone's personal identity. Vintage-aged folks tend to feel more secure with their identities, even without external definitions, reinforcements, and acknowledgements.

Consider the Possibilities

Back to the Decision Tree: the scenario that depicts the easiest possible decision is the unimpeded path to retirement, with or without a plan, but with a feeling of comfort about the decision. That decision is represented in the diagram as the first vertical set of boxes to the far left. This set of factors is a no-brainer: simple, uncomplicated, done.

However, some of us are forced into retirement through downsizing, other economy-driven factors, or by disability. Betsy, you may recall, was in her fifties when her neurologically based disability prevented her from continuing to work as a scientist. It took her about five years to recover enough strength and quell her fears about starting something new. Unfortunately, going back to science wasn't an option. When she finally came out of the fog of sickness, she used her child-like curiosity, buried deep within and untapped for decades, to explore life anew and to follow any path that seemed interesting. Reminiscing one day, she fondly recalled her long-ago and faraway summer camp experiences with art projects. Accidentally retrieving this memory invigorated and focused her exploration a bit. Laughing as she described with amazement her newfound ability to tolerate the lack of structure in her life, she watched herself plodding along without a clear path to define this phase of life—a new experience for sure and a bit uncomfortable for her at first.

Out of necessity, she had done what she likely could not have tolerated before. She suspended her need for control while trusting her instincts as never before. Perhaps a lengthy time-out caused by illness and the trauma of losing her job yielded to living comfortably one day at a time with a let's-try-this-and-see-how-it-feels attitude. Fortunately, meandering through a series of visual art forms led her to her current passion in ceramics.

The Working Artist

Though very few interviewees were still working when we spoke, that choice is certainly a viable option. The decision to not retire might be informed by numerous scenarios, some of which are outlined in the Decision Tree 1 diagram.

Scenario #1: You enjoy working or at least find that for the moment you aren't ready to stop. Maybe work is still feeding your ego, or your career started late, or there are financial considerations, or you just plain love what you do.

In that case, finding your art form will be no different a process than it would have been at any prior time in your life. That being said, incorporating a new interest will take some time, space, and discipline. But then again, being a Vintage-Years person, you already know what's required to begin something new and the well-worn patterns in your brain will guide you.

The starting point is your curiosity and openness to whatever arts you notice as you live day to day. You might start by saying to yourself, "I could do that," like Marty did as a young man visiting an art museum for the first time with his new wife. True, he didn't get started as an artist for another thirty-five years, but at least he identified an art medium that excited him.

Talk to artists of all sorts. Use this opportunity to rule in and rule out, the way you would in an informational interview to help you decide if a potential job would be a good fit for you. Any next steps will mirror what most people do to get started: take classes, buy a cheap easel and some paints, borrow or rent a guitar, or buy a notebook and start writing something just to see how it feels.

Judy, whom we met in Part II, was still working when she walked into an art gallery while vacationing on Cape Cod and found herself buying a sketch pad and watercolors about an hour later. This felt very impulsive to her, but she followed her instinct. It was the beginning of her love affair with watercolors. She was fifty-seven at the time. Though she works intermittently on a per diem basis as a hospital social worker, painting is a central element in her busy life.

Scenario #2: You no longer enjoy working but don't want to retire. Perhaps you outgrew your job, are tired of chasing new technology, or you're ready for a fresh challenge. There are all kinds of possibilities here. As Decision Tree 1 suggests, explore alternative options, such as new jobs or volunteer opportunities that might create a better fit. Consider the variety of resources listed below, first as volunteer possibilities and then as prospects for alternative paid work.

Resources and Opportunities

To help you target volunteer agencies with which to match your rich set of experiences and wisdom, consider the following:

- Experience Corps (www.experiencecorps.org) works to solve significant social problems, starting with literacy. Its age fifty-five and over members tutor and mentor urban public school children. Part of the AmeriCorps (www.americorps.gov) national service network, it supports on a yearly basis the engagement of nearly 75,000 older Americans to meet critical needs in education, the environment, public safety, homeland security, and other areas.

- Senior Corps (www.seniorcorps.org) is an online site and clearinghouse for volunteers over fifty-five. It even offers a link to job openings. A few program offerings from Senior Corps include: 1) The Foster Grandparent Program, which allows volunteers age fifty-five and older to help children and young people who have exceptional needs; 2) The Senior Companion Program, which supports adults who live in the same community as volunteers but have problems performing everyday tasks; and 3) The RSVP Program, which is for anyone over the age of fifty-five. It finds community services that match a senior's skill set. It helps seniors meet others with whom they have something in common.

- Encore Careers (www.encore.org) mobilizes the talent of fifty-five-plus individuals who want to work, not so much for the money but to "leave the world a better place than you found it." Encore taps the knowledge and energy of older adults to do what they love but in a context that benefits society in direct ways—by generally helping others in the public sector. Encore.org is published by Civic Ventures (www.civicventures.org), a nonprofit think tank focusing on baby boomers, work, and social purpose.

- Coming of Age (www.comingofage.org) has a mission to help "people fifty and older explore their future, connect and contribute through opportunities, both paid and unpaid, in their communities." Coming of Age also provides "training to nonprofits about how to build their capacity to capture the energy and expertise of this population." The dynamic website is inspirational and highlights the lives of those over fifty who have made a difference to others and organizations they serve.

The final category on Decision Tree 1 is for those who can't retire because of financial needs. The first decade of the twenty-first century was financially brutal to countless people. There is a rule of thumb in the world of economics that says that if the stock market is doing poorly within five years of your retirement, it will be difficult to make savings last through the remaining years. As I write this book, many baby boomers are struggling with a shortfall of money. If you are one of them, you can work and still give voice to your inner artist.

Will part time work meet your needs, or is full time employment still necessary? In either case, there are a few links available through the volunteer organizations listed above if you wish to make a change but need to stay in the workforce.

If you are financially challenged, getting into the arts will most closely mirror the experience of working folks highlighted in "The Working Artist" above. One disclaimer: temporarily avoid the arts that require an outlay of money for equipment or classes. I hear that oil paints are expensive, but probably not as expensive as playing golf on a regular basis.

Decision Tree 2

We approach the Vintage Years with vastly different styles, personalities, and traits. Fixed traits, such as general intelligence and genetic predispositions, are quite stable. We can't change them as much as we can work with and around them. Personalities flow out of fixed traits but are shaped by those around us, by family and friends, as well as by life experiences and the culture we reside in. Styles resemble personal preferences that are reinforced over time and become our preferred ways of seeing or interacting with the world. Our psychological and emotional qualities become imprinted onto everything we do, including our art—affecting not just *what* we choose to learn but *how*.

Note the differences: Dan's planned, systematic approach to beginning an artist's life by going back to college was a far cry from Yvette's accidental stumbling onto the writer's life by penning her first short story to reduce the boredom of a lengthy train trip along the Eastern Seaboard. Betsy was searching for something meaningful to do following her forced retirement. Her plan was to explore and stay open to possibilities that intrigued her, but she had no idea where the meandering would take her. John loved classical music and impulsively bought a grand piano for his living room when he finally settled in one place. Only later did he decide to play it himself.

Decision Tree 2 takes up where the first one trails off, focusing on the temperamental, emotional, and psychological factors that impact *how* you find and manage your art. It makes the assumption that you now have more space and time to assess how to find the meaning and enjoyment that were in short supply until this time. And, of course, you will do it entirely your own way.

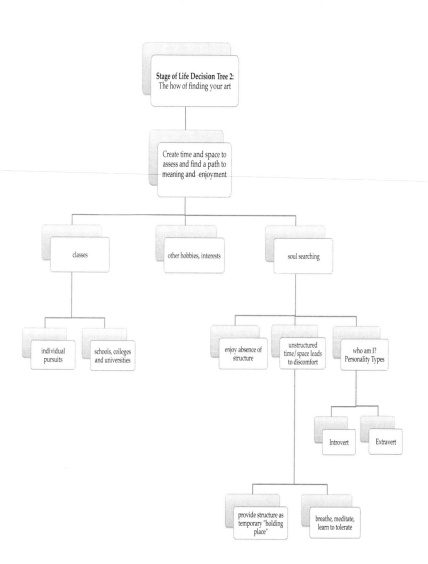

Different Strokes for Different Folks

How the artists in this book tackled the search for new options beyond work is every bit as important as *what* they chose to do or *when* they began their explorations. Some of their differences related to personality types and styles. For example, introverts and extraverts approach life in different ways. Those who tend to be more introverted, and by that I mean that they are comfortable learning and doing their art alone, follow a more solitary style. Not that they avoid people, but unlike extraverts, they don't require a large daily dose of people.

Extraverts tend to be energized by others and crave contact with others, so classes and group projects fit their needs best. But introverts need solitude to collect their thoughts and recover from the energy required by spending large chunks of time with others. Michelle, the novel writer we met in Part II, lives in a secluded wooded area and takes long walks alone to recharge her battery and gain inspiration. When she wants companionship, she makes a few phone calls or goes to a yoga class in town.

Those who are more adventuresome make different choices than homebodies. Risk takers embrace life's decisions in ways that non-risk takers wouldn't even consider. Marty, both extraverted and adventuresome, combined his first exposure to art with a weekend workshop far from home, and it was a perfect beginning. John's piano, on the other hand, anchors him to home and performing for an audience of one. That's the way he likes it.

Structure versus absence of structure is another factor worth considering. As you can see from Decision Tree 2, soul searching has at least three components. Some folks can't wait to wake up in the morning without a plan and then see what develops. Retirement without structure is perfect for their style. Following the death of her 107-year-old mother, Caroline needed the freedom to just live life on a daily basis exactly as it presented itself. It took three years before a plan for her writing hobby emerged. The space and time didn't make her the least bit anxious. If that characterizes you, no need to consider the other options.

But if open space and time without punctuation makes you uncomfortable, you have different options as you move forward. You can put a temporary plan in place as a holding structure, or you can learn to tolerate the discomfort. While the first choice is a lot easier, it does require an additional step. Still, it's a kind of security blanket that protects you from the feeling of having walked off a cliff after the retirement party ends.

I've heard from so many people that not being busy is a fearsome idea. Why not just make it easier for yourself by inventing next steps and then discarding them if they don't live up to your expectations or as they are no longer necessary. It took Eileen a while to find her passion in photography, but she didn't wait until it called her name. She started with painting and over time fine-tuned her interest.

Julie's retirement coincided with her father's death, leaving two giant holes to fill. Wanting to keep herself busy, she jumped headlong into church activities that bolstered her confidence and increased her outgoingness. At that point she was ready to take on something new and challenging. "Indeed, I took my first drawing class in February 1999. It was appealingly called, 'I've Never Held a Pencil: A Very Basic Drawing Class.' The teacher was perfect, and I was hooked."

An alternative to getting busy is to manage the discomfort of not knowing what's next. Create space to think without discomfort. Easier said than done? There's probably no better tool than meditation. In its simplest form, it requires no more than sitting and noticing your breathing. You can get fancy and find all kinds of classes: mindfulness, Buddhist styles, and several kinds of yoga. Any of these practices will be a good choice if you enjoy being around other like-minded people. On the other hand, and for more introverted readers, just sit and breathe for fifteen or twenty minutes, catching your attention when it wanders and bringing it back to your breath. This gives you something to *do*, if your personal style necessitates it, without running headlong into the first hobby that promises to fill a void.

In the end, it's important to know yourself and what you need to make your life both comfortable and interesting. Get to know and appreciate your personality traits, habits and quirks. It will be more than helpful in your retirement decision-making process and in finding your art.

Finally, keep in mind that the process is virtually the same whether you choose to write, to paint, or to play a musical instrument. Even if you broaden your horizons to include learning a craft or beginning to play bridge or mahjong, the process of *how* you approach it is the same. This strategy also applies to other projects that encompass newness, problem solving, and complexity, the triumvirate that most contributes to brain activity and sustained growth.

10 Bravo to the Life Well Lived

Our truest life is when we are in dreams awake.
—Henry David Thoreau

Hooray to all who discovered passion through the expression of their art in the last third of life. We've had a chance to peek into the decision-making and daily routines of more than twenty fine artists of all kinds. Their stories, while unique, have at least three points in common: 1) Their youthful years didn't support or reinforce the artistic potential we are all born with and is hardwired into our species; 2) Young adulthood and middle adulthood did nothing to reward any of their efforts to adopt an art form. Maybe they had a brief flirtation with learning the guitar or taking a ceramics course, but the demands of adulthood, reinforced by society, made art a nearly impossible option; and, 3) The Vintage Years ushered in a personal Renaissance, a golden age of artistry for all of them.

As we consolidate what we know about the Vintage Years and review the confluence of factors that facilitate the emergence of our inner artist, I offer yet another story about an octogenarian who's name may be familiar or who's work may have made a difference in your life. His life story provides a final example of the artistic accomplishments possible in the Vintage Years.

One More Artist's Story

In 1938, to avoid Hitler's European expansion and aggression, a sixteen-year-old Jewish lad named Carl Djerassi escaped from Vienna. As the story goes, he arrived in the U.S. penniless but yearning for a college education. In his naivety and with the belief that the U.S. was a place where anything was possible, he sent a letter to Eleanor Roosevelt asking her to help him find a scholarship. To the amazement of others, her secretary found a scholarship for him to a college from which he graduated summa cum laude at eighteen.

Most of us don't have experiences that resemble Carl's early life. Still, like the rest of us, achievement, marriage, family, and a profession marked his middle years. Following the traditional route of scholars, albeit at a much faster pace, he completed a Ph.D. in chemistry at the ripe old age of twenty-two and embarked on a brilliant and successful career.

He is best known as the "father of the birth control pill," which in 1961 greatly changed contraception practices in the U.S. and Europe. Fitting very well into the role of scientist, researching, publishing his findings, and teaching absorbed his energies during the mid-section of his life. The details of his professional accomplishments are well documented in other books and articles; therefore I'm concentrating on his transformation into a writer at sixty.

I exchanged e-mails with Dr. Djerassi. Now in his late eighties, he has quite a robust schedule. He divides his time between two continents doing public speaking about his writing and providing a retreat in California for mentoring young writers. He suggested that he covered all of my interview questions in great detail in several chapters of one of his books. So I turned to his writing and learned about the impetus that fueled his poetry and later novel and play writing.

He wrote, "The love of my life . . . announced with a tender thunderbolt that she had fallen in love with another man." As you might expect, Carl's reaction, in his own words, was "humorless, self pitying, (with) the urge for revenge." Swimming in a sea of emotions ranging from sadness to rage, a lifeline finally presented itself. "The surprise was an outpouring of poems—confessional, self pitying, and even narcissistic. It was a cathartic experience for someone who until then had never written a single line of verse."[48]

His poetry writing continued but his bitterness subsided. "As the number of my published poems grew, I started to take myself seriously . . . . I was sensible enough to recognize that it was too late in life to turn into a real poet; I realized that the chief value of this lyrical outpouring was therapeutic[49]." Carl then turned to novel writing. His first attempt served the purpose of giving full expression to his pain and suffering and "demonstrated that I possessed a writer's discipline."

Subsequently, getting back together with the love of his life, he tried writing short stories first before tackling another work of fiction. A summer stay in England gave him time to write and led to a series of short stories, eleven exactly, which were com-

---

[48] *This Man's Pill*, pp. 137–138

[49] p. 143

bined to form his first published book of fiction. A second novel emerged the following summer.

While his motivation to write wasn't exactly clear to me, his own words suggested that "these fishing expeditions into my unconscious started to teach me a great deal about myself, and of course this fascinated me. Scientists are on the whole not self-reflective. I certainly never was. But as I started to examine what made me tick, my stories started to assume a psychoanalytical resonance."[50] It's probably no accident that Carl's introspection emerged during his Vintage Years which we now know fosters the process of looking inward without the drama of testosterone-driven emotion more characteristic of younger adulthood.

Carl segued into something he called "science in fiction" writing, to be distinguished from science fiction, as a way to bring science to the masses. Becoming a scientist-turned-author allowed him to introduce the public to science in a user-friendly way by telling stories that just happen to include science. The reception to his novel, *Cantor's Dilemma*, an example of the science-in-fiction genre, ". . . encouraged me to lock the door of my laboratory from the outside and throw away the key."[51]

He comments that writing about aging scientists and the dilemma of their retirement made him "wonder about my own dismissive attitude toward voluntary retirement. Was it pride or just a manifestation of a workaholic's machismo?"[52] Once again, this is an age-appropriate task or struggle, and its resolution is a

---

[50] p. 154

[51] p. 167

[52] Ibid.

hallmark of the Vintage Years. His writing allowed and even facilitated the process of slogging through his feelings about retirement. Still, I don't know if retirement is the word I would use to describe the next twenty-five years of Carl's life. Yes, he closed his lab and stopped teaching, but he morphed into a passionate and dedicated writer.

Carl Djerassi, eighty-nine at the time of this writing, is still going strong. First he wrote poems, then novels, and finally plays—what a prolific artist. He set the stage for his later life and realized his lasting goal: to bring science to the non-scientist in an understandable and palatable form.

Is this an example of a legacy desire to leave something valuable behind or is it perhaps related more to generativity, the process of using one's knowledge to mentor and benefit society through wisdom? Maybe one or the other, maybe both. Carl is manifesting several of the Vintage Years urges we've already explored, not because he read the book but because these are the developmental tasks of the sixty-plus years. Bravo Carl, for a full and meaningful life still unfolding!

Act Three

Very few artists get it right the first time, with a few exceptions like Mozart. And so it makes sense that the third iteration of just about anything is often the best. Similarly, the third act of life benefits from all our experiences and practice, enhanced with wisdom—a quality that by definition can't manifest before the Vintage Years. This time frame is like a crescendo, when diverse and seemingly disparate forces and events, not particularly profound in and of themselves, come together and create an outcome that could only happen at that point in time and because of that combination of factors. What manifests is greater than the sum of its constituent parts, a synergistic process.

While talking about the confluence of contributory factors that inform the Vintage Years, I decided to make a formula out of it, the way Gene Cohen created his formula, $C=me^2$. To refresh your memory, his equation "represents the ultimate synergy of the multiple facets of our creativity equation: the mass of material that you have accrued in a given body of knowledge and of your 'e' outer world experience and inner 'e' world experience." He uses this formula to demonstrate how creative potential increases as we age and as we "explore new areas of interest and new forms of expression."[53]

The formula I suggest is a summation of the following factors: the child's artistic curiosity (a), plus hormonal changes in late adulthood (h), plus accumulated life experience (l), plus brain laterality and plasticity (b), plus free time (f), plus increased meaning and legacy (m), plus wisdom (w), plus awareness of mortality (aom). Altogether, they explain the increased potential for artistic expression after the age of sixty (ipae>60) in this nifty formula: $a+h+l+b+f+m+w+aom=ipae>60$.

The good news about this formula is that you don't have to memorize it. Why? Because you are actually capable of *living it right now*. And that is this book's central thesis. Add together the equation's elements and the stage is set for your increased capacity to write a book or to start playing the guitar or to create an art object. Of course, doing these things requires patience and practice time, but fortunately patience and time are more abundantly available in the Vintage Years than at any other time in life.

---

[53] *The Creative Age*, p. 110

Finding My Inner Artist

I had my own questions about the Vintage Years, which prompted an exploration that eventually became a book. That was before the word *vintage* came to define a life stage. My impulsive decision at seventy to rent a cello, without the foggiest idea about how I would learn to play it, was based on a video I found online. I am most grateful for Biana Kovic's work with older cello students, which gave me some small hope that I might still be capable of learning.

It's no accident that this epiphany coincided with my decision to retire from practice as a clinical psychologist. After forty-five years of being deeply immersed in all aspects of my profession, I thought it was time, as Cozolino wrote about so eloquently, to explore what still might be left to do to complete my life.

Finding a wonderful cello teacher who, to my surprise, was not the least bit daunted by my age turned out to be the first step after lugging my rented cello home in its rented case. It helped that my teacher was herself north of sixty years old. This wasn't an accident; I ruled out candidates who might be too young to understand the power of over-sixty intentionality and passion. It helped that she was also the principal cellist with a big city opera company. As I saw it, if I was going to be serious and with time running out, I'd best find a teacher who walked the walk and could inspire me to greatness. Not that I've achieved greatness, mind you. That wasn't my aspiration nor does it fit with my goals for the Vintage Years.

After eighteen months of weekly lessons and daily practice for forty minutes per day, divided into two twenty-minute segments, I am capable of playing beautiful music, at least to my ears! Consistent with what I know about adult learning, and especially learning as an older adult, it's best to have spaced learning: short daily practice sessions over a long period of time. Cramming is for the young! The older adult needs many repetitions to reinforce short-term memory so that it can convert to long-term memory. Fortunately, I now have the time and generally the patience for this slower process to unfold.

Writing is also part of my daily habit, and I find to my great delight that writing seems to bypass some of the difficulty I have retrieving words when I'm speaking. I am more fluent with my written language than my spoken language. This is a pleasant happenstance that certainly makes me want to write more and talk less! No one in my circle seems to mind or maybe even notice.

I write for all the same reasons as other Vintage Years folks who fill notebooks of paper or generate pages on digital devices. Also, like other psychologists who write, I wish to add to the body of knowledge about how the brain accommodates change in the last third of life because it has personal relevance. Finally, I wish to hand forward to a new generation whatever small bits of wisdom I like to think I've accumulated as the years passed and which hopefully serve as part of my legacy.

The Vintage Season of the Mind

Elkhonon Goldberg, Ph.D., was fifty-eight and a neuropsychologist when he wrote about wisdom. "The feeling that 'the seasons of our mind' are not all downhill and that some important mental gains are attained as we age is grounded in neurobiological reality; it is not merely a desperate exercise in wishful thinking by an aging intellectual.... Those of us whose mental lives have been both vigorous and rigorous approach their advanced years with a mighty coat of mental armor.... This mental armor, the rich collection of pattern-recognizing attractors in the brain, is not an entitlement and its attainment in old age is not a foregone conclusion. It is a reward for the vigorous life of the mind in younger years. "[54]

Based on Goldberg's prescription, I continue playing the cello and writing. I alternate time with each of these art forms and top it off with daily exercise, as John Ratey, M.D., author of *Spark,* suggests. According to him, "Exercise sparks connections and growth among your brain's cell networks. It increases blood volume, regulates fuel, and encourages neuronal activity and neurogenesis."[55] It is "the single most powerful tool you have to optimize your brain function."[56] Ratey is not alone in this. Over and over, the psychological and neuroscience literature acknowledges the connection between physical exercise and brain vitality.

The Strength of Social Connections

What else can we add to the mix in order to optimize the conditions for learning and to maintain the brain in tip-top shape? The importance of our social networks, particularly as we age, is implied throughout this book and illustrated in the artists' stories in Part II, but I feel that it needs to be made even more

---

[54] p. 288

[55] p. 223

[56] p. 245

explicit. The narratives of the artists I interviewed overlapped in still one other significant way: their emerging-artist lifestyle brought new people, activities, and ideas into their lives in abundance.

Everyone reported a sense of comradery with the others they met while doing their art in classes, workshops, and studios. Barbara, the African drummer, talked about meeting other drummers whose lifestyles were so different from hers that it was unlikely she would ever have encountered them if not through music camps and various drumming gigs. She appreciates the broadened perspective they brought to the way she looks at life.

Our social connections and engagements are particularly important in later years as loved ones and old friends begin to move on in one way or another. New friends, new ideas, new activities, and new cues resulting from going to places that only your art takes you, including outside of your comfort zone, all stimulate the brain. Remember that novelty, complexity, and problem solving comprise the triumvirate that stokes the engine of the brain, increasing neuronal production, enhancing brain reserve, and strengthening the immune system that supports overall good health. The arts serve as the perfect mechanism for fostering social connections.

Revisiting the Core Ideas

This book began with my curiosity about: 1) how artistic expression stimulates the aging brain; and 2) how the aging brain facilitates artistic expression.

Let's first review how artistic expression stimulates the aging brain. The arts help to keep and build the brain's robustness in the last third of life, and the Vintage Years provide the perfect venue for creativity to emerge in one or more forms.

The new science of creativity, according to Jonah Lehrer, author of "How to be Creative,"[57] supports the idea that creativity is a learned skill and not inherited. Creativity requires hard work plus time to think, to daydream, or to try out various combinations of whatever one is trying to generate. It also requires less self-consciousness and fear of failure as well as a reduction of inhibition, which Lehrer says comes with age. This sounds a lot like childhood to me.

According to Albert Einstein, who had something to say about this as well, "Everything that is really great and inspiring is created by the individual who can labor in freedom."[58] The Vintage Years provide the ultimate laboratory where freedom to manifest creativity is possible, where creativity can freely bubble up and find expression. This is a stage in life when time is most plentiful and the stress associated with getting things done is minimal—the perfect combination to stimulate creativity. While this book focuses on the fine arts as a conduit to building brain strength, there certainly are other ways to increase novelty, complexity and problem solving.

A good friend, recently retired and perhaps influenced by his wife who is a bridge player, decided to take up bridge. While I don't play myself, I am told that each and every hand requires problem solving; the recognition of a complex set of patterns. My friend was trained as a physicist, but studying bridge gives

---

[57] *The Wall Street Journal*, March 10, 2012

[58] Saying attributed to Einstein.

his brain a good workout, according to him—so much so that his daily routine requires hours of study bordering on frustrating but always invigorating.

There are many other hobbies that serve as brain tonics. While writing this book, I was approached by Vintage-aged folks who are creative gardeners, scrap bookers, and golfers, to name a few, making their case for the artistry associated with their endeavors. There's no doubt that these pastimes are stimulating and can help the brain's neurogenesis. Why then did I limit my study to visual arts, music, and writing?

Why the Fine Arts?

The more I researched, the more I was convinced that the fine arts do in fact continue to have the survival value that anthropologists and evolutionary biologists and psychologists suggest was true in the dawn of humankind. Receptivity to art continues to be something that humans value and experience with pleasure, even passion. There is evidence that expressing art increases dopamine production in the brain, which in turn increases the experience of pleasure and the good feelings that are often associated with certain addictive drugs.

As detailed in Chapter 2, young children everywhere come to the arts naturally only to drift away or to be dissuaded when time and talent don't appear in abundance. A long stretch of adulthood follows with some nostalgia for an art that was attempted and abandoned earlier or never attempted at all. Early and middle adulthood are not usually conducive to art exploration.

Take the case of Gary Marcus, Ph.D., the author of *Guitar Zero*, whom we met in the introduction to Part II: "My only realistic

hope of learning to play an instrument was to become completely immersed.... I figured that I had no more chance of becoming
musical by playing three minutes every other week than I had of
learning to fly."[59] Marcus clearly understood that it would take
consistent effort and many months, in his case a year and a half,
to play the guitar to his minimal satisfaction. Because it was during the adulthood stage of life, a time-out from his day job was
required to seriously pursue musical practice. Thankfully, his
sabbatical year gave him a head start for the time and focus he
needed to begin.

One of the conclusions he came to was that "music, as we
have seen, is more like a lifelong journey than a few weeks' project, more like chess than checkers. Although many of the
rudiments of music fit naturally with the human mind, master-
ing the detail is an ongoing project."[60] Since most of us don't
have a sabbatical year to devote to learning an art form, our artistic yearnings generally need to wait for the Vintage Years.

A friend of mine in her late fifties is an accomplished scientist
with both M.D. and Ph.D. degrees. We spoke about my book
when it was still an embryonic project, and she wistfully reported that she had always wanted to play the piano. She spoke as if
that could no longer happen. Mind you, she wasn't talking about
becoming a concert pianist but someone who could play well
enough to entertain herself and feel the passion of playing music. Yet she thought about it like an impossible dream whose
time had passed. Jokingly, I suggested that she read my book

---

[59] p. 11

[60] p. 35

when I finished writing it because she could indeed make that dream a reality; she was approaching the one time in life when musical expression had a high likelihood of really happening for her. I reminded her that, changes in the brain beginning at mid-life actually help the new artist. This was the second idea that piqued my curiosity when I began to think about writing this book: how the aging brain facilitates artistic expression.

How the Aging Brain Facilitates Artistic Expression

Let's review what happens to the brain, beginning in midlife that actually helps with learning to sculpt, play the piano, or write a novel. There is plentiful evidence that the older brain functions at least as well as the young or middle-aged brain in most ways except for speed of analyzing data.

According to Michael Sweeney, Ph.D., author of *Brain: The Complete Mind, How it Develops, How it Works and How to Keep it Sharp*, "It may move more slowly, but it moves with greater purpose. Except for a decrease in processing speed, the healthy mature brain performs about as well as a youthful one in any task requiring planning, analysis, and organization of infor-mation. And with the wisdom of a lifetime, the elderly brain usually out performs the youthful brain in judgment."[61]

While scientific evidence is just beginning to corroborate the idea that the Vintage Years are ideally suited for learning, the societal bias toward youth is slow to change. Making a case to explain elder art ability would not be necessary at all if it were not for the youth-idolizing culture of the West, including the

---

[61] p. 267

United States. I personally think that the diversity of cultural influences in the U.S.—especially a century of immigration from Asia where elders are highly valued—has had very beneficial effects.

Though changing perceptions toward aging is a slow process, it is beginning to happen, fueled in part by the U.S. baby-boomer generation coming of age: youthful, demanding to be taken seriously, and determined to remain vibrant.

As seniors push for more respect, the scientific community has taken greater notice and allocated more financial resources to study the healthy aging brain. This confluence has resulted in more sophisticated ways of studying the brain using the new neuroimaging techniques described earlier. The fMRI and PET study the brain in real time, looking at what is actually happening when it is engaged in thinking and problem solving. Other brain mapping techniques focus on brain structures and their changes. All in all, neuroscientists have at their disposal a number of cutting-edge research tools to understand more than ever how the brain works and changes as a result of aging or disease.

Through current research efforts, we are beginning to accumulate some evidence of positive changes in the brain that facilitate the new artist's attempts to learn. For example:

1) Bilaterality: During youth and adulthood, the hallmark of the left hemisphere is its ability to process linear, logical, and sequential information. The right hemisphere is involved in emotional regulation, imagination, and the processing of visual images. Novelty is mostly dealt with in the right hemisphere, but once the problem is under-

stood or solved, the left hemisphere becomes engaged and is the site from which it is retrieved as a learned pattern.

Starting at midlife, the right and left hemispheres of the brain become better integrated, more interdependent and functionally intertwined. The right hemisphere becomes less effective in learning and holding new information, a normal and natural consequence of aging. The left hemisphere compensates with its rich patterning ability. At this point, both sides of the brain may be used to perform the same task—and two sides are superior to one! Also, thoughts and feelings are now better united than at any previous life stage.

2) Patterning: Let's review Elkhonon Goldberg's words about the right-to-left-hemisphere shift as we age. "The left hemisphere is of foremost importance in mature years, the season of wisdom, of seeing new things through the prism of vast past experience," and the left hemisphere "accumulates an ever-increasing 'library' of efficient pattern-recognition devices in the form of neural attractors."[62]

Patterning, a shorthand process that is most robust in the later years, allows a huge number of learned ideas to come together in new combinations. This may account for the creativity in the later years, the ability to draw upon a vast storehouse of lifelong learning to be expressed in unique, fresh, and complex ways.

3) Hormones: You may recall that we spoke of the decrease in estrogen and testosterone in the years between fifty and sixty. In both men and women, the biologically-driven

---

[62] p. 214

urges of competition and emotionally-driven decision making and judgments give way to greater emotional stability, calmness, and increased focus of attention. This change results in greater patience and increased tolerance for frustration, significantly benefitting the study of fine arts.

Coming Full Circle

This book wouldn't be complete without an update about Biana Kovic, the New York City cello teacher whose DVD *Virtuoso* got me thinking about playing the cello in the first place. Biana and I talked recently, five years after her video was published. Of course, I was curious about Matty Kahn, who began her study of the cello at eighty-nine and recently turned ninety-five.

Matty continued to take weekly lessons with Biana following the six-week, five-time-per-week, intensive instruction period that was captured in the DVD. She intended to play the cello indefinitely and regained some lost vitality—both physically and emotionally, according to Biana. "Matty was lonely when I met her. Her life had lost meaning. She had lost touch, the physical sensation of being close with something or someone," which Matty said she got from being with the cello. Biana went on, "You know, you hold it next to your body and you have the feeling you are holding someone. She felt like her whole body was changing because of that experience. She started to feel better about herself. Learning the cello changed Matty's concept of what was appropriate to do at her age." It so inspired her that she revisited the visual arts, previously important in her life, with renewed enthusiasm. A flurry of pastels and paintings resulted. At ninety-one, she was "named the Judge's Choice Award winner in the 2008 NY Coo Open Art Contest for her painting, 'The Breath of the Sunflower.'"[63]

Regarding her cello playing, after several months of lessons, Matty had an accident resulting in a lengthy recuperation and she hasn't resumed lessons. Still, the time she spent learning a musical instrument and expressing her satisfaction and passion through it shaped her early nineties and remains with her as a source of increased pride and self-esteem.

Biana summed up the experience of taking art seriously in the later years. Her own father was a sculptor hobbyist who kept producing pieces even when their home was running out of space to display them. When she asked her father why he kept at it, he referred to it as "auto-legacy:" giving back to himself, taking the pleasure and meaning infused in his art and giving himself a gift of it, recognizing and appreciating "with enormous pride his own greatness, his own existence." I think this must be true for all Vintage Years artists to some extent—finding and bathing in the joy that comes with being immersed in the art that nurtures in return.

---

[63] *The Riverdale Press*, March 18, 2008

Afterword

As *The Vintage Years* took it's final form and the home stretch was almost visible, two major events happened that led to this Afterword. One was personal and the other was awe-inspiring.

The first event gave me the opportunity to put into practice some of the lessons I absorbed from the many artists I had the privilege to interview. I heard their words of support and encouragement in my head when I wondered how I would handle some serious and negative health news out of left field.

With one chapter left to write I learned that I had lung cancer, a shocking piece of news that threatened not just my timeline but also my life. The numerous tests to determine the extent, prognosis and treatment seemed to take forever as time seemed altered and played in slow motion. It provided an opportunity to review my life as it had been and life as it might unfold or lead to an abrupt halt.

News like this doesn't make any sense when you are a nonsmoker. There's no way to explain it but there are ways to manage it. The initial uncertainty required my psychologist skills to imagine various scenarios, not only the worst-case situations with catastrophic outcomes. I knew it would be way too easy to focus on morose thoughts if my emotions and thoughts followed the path of least resistance. So I chose to live the artist's way—to practice my art every day as much as possible both to distract myself from fantasizing about the unknown and to write the last chapter of this book. I also continued playing the cello as if nothing had changed.

The *good* news received later was that surgery was an option that could lead to a possible full recovery. The *bad* news was that surgery was necessary to remove a tumor and a lobe from my lung. I played the cello and wrote madly late into the night preceding the day of surgery, finishing the last chapter. Luckily the surgery went optimally.

As I write this Afterword six months later I've resumed all of my former activities, living each day fully, grateful for learning to be so totally involved in writing and playing music that I did experience time-outs from worry and pain. Thankfully, the future looks bright and timeless again.

The other major event that occurred after I thought I'd completed *The Vintage Years* was meeting Tim Carpenter, the creator of the Burbank Senior Artists' Colony where people like those in the book live together and embody what this book is all about.

His concept was novel and when he made it real, it was so popular that several other projects based on his Burbank model sprung to life. When Tim and I met in Burbank I heard his passion and saw the evidence of his dream. For me, it served as tangible evidence that taking up an art form, whether painting or collage, playing the trumpet or guitar, writing plays and/or acting in them, all contribute to well being and satisfaction for the over fifty-five population. The added bonus of living together with other artists, creating synergy and stimulating the brain, testify to the practice that I preached.

Tim is not a senior citizen, not even close, which made me curious about his interest in the creativity of elders. He began working in the senior housing field in the late '90s and told me that after his first visit to a senior apartment complex, "What I saw was a blank canvas because no one was doing anything cool whatsoever." With a background as a writer and playwright he could see the possibilities. "I'm going to start a writing class because I can teach it," he thought in his pragmatic style. His goal was "to bring a college lifestyle to retirement." My tour of the Burbank Senior Artist's Colony reminded me of a busy college campus with students, albeit grey haired and without skateboards, rushing to classes carrying canvases, instruments and notebooks.

What makes Tim's model totally unique is the focus on affordable housing; bringing the arts to seniors living on social security and modest incomes. This is a population often ignored because the expression of art is not generally thought to be a basic need like food or shelter even though as we've seen in The Vintage Years, it really does have primacy and was part of our primordial past.

Tim saw the potential for all seniors, not just the ones who could afford private instruction. "I wanted this to be in the inner city not up on the hill ... bringing it here where they live and providing it for free, so that you can walk downstairs and be engaged." Tim realized the pun, *engAGE* , which is the name of his non-profit, as he reflected on the past ten years.

This live-in-art model is also one of immersion, different from Elderhostel, for example, which may introduce seniors to art expression but only for a weekend or a week. Tim and I agreed that older folks don't learn well by cramming and do best with learning over time, preferably on a daily basis. Clearly, living where you do your art, surrounded by those also immersed in what they love, creates the ideal learning environment.

We talked about the social, community aspects of the Burbank Center and how this is so critical to the vibrancy of older adults. "You have to leave room for the magic thing to happen because telling people doesn't work, they need to see it for themselves." Living among budding artists provides inspiration and fantastic role modeling. Tim's vision, living together and making art, builds on his earliest memories "I grew up near an artist colony in upstate New York called Yaddo. It had a profound impact on me." Little did he know then that he would later incorporate the artist colony lifestyle into his life's work with seniors.

Happily, this idea is spreading with Tim planting the seeds in local non-profits around California and elsewhere to duplicate his model based on local community needs. To learn more about what Tim Carpenter is up to at *engAGE*, you can go to the URL: www.engagedaging.org.

Certain that the Senior Artist Colony story would be the last, *The Vintage Years* headed for a final review and tying together a few loose ends.

Taking a lunch break with a friend led to a chance meeting with her brother-in-law and still another tale of post-sixty artistic discovery. It's a truly remarkable account—how he found his operatic baritone voice quite accidentally after a chance encounter with a former opera singer turned coach.

Realizing that this book could go on endlessly as I continue to meet men and women who've found their inner artist during this life stage, I decided to save their accounts for the sequel!

Appendix: Artists' Work

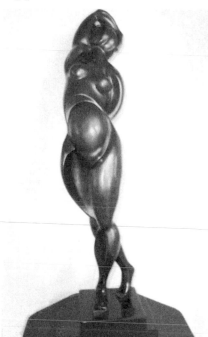

Left:

Bronze sculpture by Marty

Below:

Julie's botanical watercolor

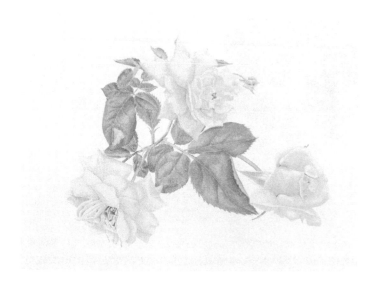

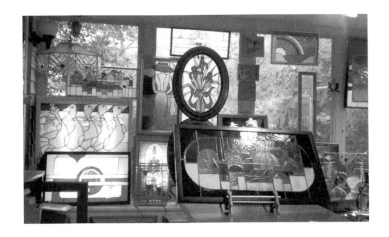

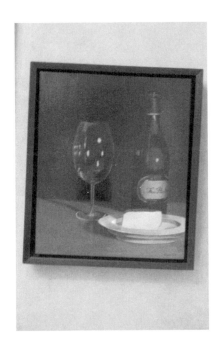

Above:

Harold's stained glass workshop

Left:

A still life painting by Dan

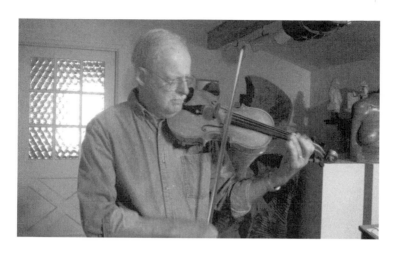

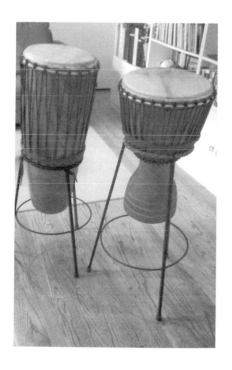

Above:

Don playing the fiddle he made in his music and art studio.

Left:

Barbara's African drums

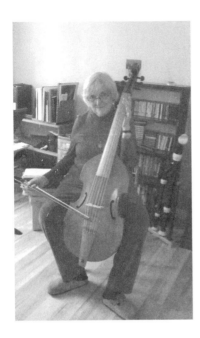

Left:

Charmion with her Viola da Gamba

Below:

Harold at the organ

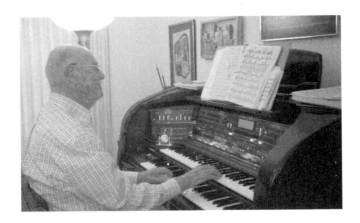

Writer's excerpts:

Essay: *Why I Write*

"Where did we come from? How did we come into being? What forces created us? These are the big questions theoretical physicists attempt to answer when they study the mystery of the Universe.

Using imagination and memory, I write about my life in an attempt to answer the same questions. Whether seeking a complete theory of the creation of the Universe or exploring the evolution of a single life, conclusions are elusive and unprovable. It doesn't matter that full understanding is unlikely. The search is its own reward.

I write for the pure joy of it—the joy of discovering what I have to say, of writing a sentence that sings, of finding the perfect word or metaphor. I write to find and record the extraordinary embedded in the ordinary. I write to surprise myself.

I write to know who I am, to identify the forces that shaped me. I write to figure out the story I'm in and to transform my splintered experiences into a whole. I write to make meaning, to understand and share my story. I write to find out what I think.

I write to forget and distance myself from difficult times and individuals. Writing offers relief from the pain of tragic events. Writing helps me forgive.

I write to remember, to honor my mother and father. I write to let family and friends know their special place in my world. I tell the stories of those who can't. I write to preserve moments of ecstasy and manage terror. I write so that others will know something of the now-vanished world that I grew up in, the same reason I keep artifacts from the fifties and sixties in my garage. I write to save. I save because I have lost. I write so that something remains.

Not unlike a scientist, I go about my work. I am on a quest. I restore the past, attend to the memories that shimmer or disturb and to the strings of memories attached to them. I roll the mind camera on vivid, life-altering moments. I deduce. I explain. I zoom out to scan for connections, themes, forces. I test conclusions for emotional truth. The work feels theoretical. I don't know where I'm going until I arrive. The process is one of discovery. I do this for myself. But I keep others in mind—the loved ones, whose stories are intertwined with mine, and strangers who might appreciate the ways in which our lives are different and the same."

—Kathleen ©

Poem: *Books, Books, Books*

"Don't give me words that ebb and flow,
    Get to the heart of what I need to know
I lose my focus when I read a tale
    That goes off on a tangent—I just lose the trail
He moved to Kentucky at age twenty-four
    After leaving the service—it was the Air Corps.

His wife took a lover, so he shot her dead
   In France he'd be knighted, they fried him instead.
I don't need three hundred pages with what they were wearing
   And the weather was misty and her bed clothes were daring.
Real life's a short story about two pages long,
   Why write all that flab with a dance and a song
You're born, you learn, you work, you wed
   You have kids, lose hair, grow old, then you're dead.
What are the chances you'll become a spy
   Or work for the president or the FBI?
If lightning strikes you will your mind increase
   So that you speak Latin, and Sanskrit and sing Portuguese?
The hero's a loafer, his wife is a slut,
   His mother's a bookie, his father's a nut.
That kind of story is clear as a bell,
   In only four lines, we know the folks well.
So save all that paper, and publishing stuff,
   Keep it simple. Concise- enough is enough!

—Yvette ©

Two Haikus:

gleaming salmon's leap
not quite high enough to clear
the third fish ladder

beyond our mailbox
the uphill road vanishes
into winter rain

—Anne ©

Acknowledgements

A book project is never a solo endeavor. Even at the conception stage, my decision to write The Vintage Years was shaped by Otis Haschemeyer, the Stanford University nonfiction creative writing teacher who plucked this idea from a number of likely suspects that were milling around in my mind. His guidance at the beginning was invaluable.

I prefer solitude when I write and much of the book spilled from my head, through my fingers and into a word document before anyone else was privy to what I was writing, except for my trusted emotional and intellectual partner, Joe Hustein, my husband who seems to know exactly what I want to say even when I can't even formulate the ideas well enough to communicate them in any form. He put up with a lot of late night reading, always patient and gentle in his critiques. I'm very grateful for his mentoring on this book, as well as the two that preceded it and actually for everything that I write.

As the rambling took on a more cogent form and most of the first draft was written I turned to my friend, fellow psychologist and professional editor, Judi Larson, Ph.D. whose low key, sometimes humorous, and smooth but firm edits immensely improved the manuscript. She provided reassurance when I started to doubt myself and reinforced my efforts by being available just when I needed her.

As things began to pull together and the manuscript sprouted a table of contents and chapter subheadings I sought the wisdom of several of my mental health colleagues and experts in the field who I could trust to read the manuscript with sharp eyes but kind hearts. Their observations, suggestions and attention to detail helped to further define, clarify and clean up the pages. Many thanks to: Heidi Ernst, M.D., Ph.D., Barbara Kirsch, Ph.D., Melanie Mopsick, LCSW, Alberta Nassi, Ph.D., Carol Schneider, Ph.D., Nancy Wesson, Ph.D., and Tamar Wishnatzky, Ed.D. Special thanks to my neuropsychologist colleagues who helped me interpret the neuroscience literature: Anders Greenwood, Ph.D., Alice Ruzicka, Ph.D., and Teresa Bailey, Ph.D. who also introduced me to the Scottish Fiddler's Association which in turn brought some very interesting late-blooming musicians to my attention. Golijeh Golarai, Ph.D., neuroscience professor at Stanford University, provided big-picture observations from her unique perspective.

Three special cellists influenced my thinking, feeling about music and the cello. They played a key role in making this book a reality. Biana Kovic, the New York City cello teacher who produced and directed the award winning documentary, Virtuoso, provided personal inspiration that sparked and fueled my interest in writing this book. Lucinda Breed Lenicheck, principal cello, Opera San Jose, California, teaches me to play the cello and translate the symbols on the written page into sounds that are pleasing, to me at least. She understands the needs of an adult learner and for that I am grateful. Over the past ten years I've had the privilege to listen up close to David Finckel, cellist with the Emerson String Quartet and co-director of Chamber Music at Lincoln Center, New York City. During the three-week summer music institute called Music@Menlo held in Menlo Park, California, of which he is the co-artistic director, he greatly influenced my decision to take up the study of the cello without even knowing it. Not only did he set the standard of excellence and passion but his mini lectures and on-line mini lessons also served to teach when I needed motivation or instruction.

Flynne and Matthew, my extraordinary adult-kids were inspirational without taking a direct role in either writing or editing. Their love and devotion have always served as a steady beacon of light energizing and nourishing my life and my writing.

And finally I wish to acknowledge and thank the many late-blooming artists I had to pleasure to interview. I can't begin to express the exhilaration and excitement that each meeting provided. These generous men and women opened their homes, studios and hearts to share their life stories with candor. They trusted that I would tell their stories fairly, capturing their love for the art that was finally free to blossom, and let it shine through the pages of this book. I hope I earned that trust. They expanded my world, added immensely to my knowledge and enriched my life more than they can imagine.

References

Cabeza, R., Lyberg, L. & Park, D. (Eds.). (2009). *Cognitive Neuroscience of Aging: Linking Cognitive and Cerebral Aging.* New York: Oxford University Press.

Cohen, G. (2006). *The Mature Mind: The Positive Power of the Aging Brain.* New York: Basic Books.

Cohen, G. (2001). *The Creative Age: Awakening Human Potential in the Second Half of Life.* New York: Quill Publishers.

Cozolino, L. (2008). *The Healthy Aging Brain.* New York: W. W. Norton & Company, Inc.

Csikszentmihalyi, M. (1993). *A Psychology for the Third Millenni um: The Evolving Self.* New York: Harper-Collins.

Csikszentmihalyi, M. (1990). *Flow: The Psychology of Optimal Experience.* New York: Harper & Row Publishers.

Delbanco, N. (2011). *Lastingness: The Art of Old Age.* New York: Grand Central Publishing.

Djerassi, C. (2004). *This Man's Pill: Reflections on the 50th Birthday of the Pill.* New York: Oxford University Press.

Djerassi, C. (1989). *Cantor's Dilemma: A Novel.* New York: Penguin Books.

Doidge, N. (2007). *The Brain That Changes Itself.* New York: Penguin Books.

Doidge, N. (2010). Interview with Allan Gregg on *Science Fri day*; TV Ontario.

Gladwell, M. (2009). *What the Dog Saw: And Other Adventures.* New York: Little, Brown & Company.

Gladwell, M. (2002). *The Tipping Point: How Little Things Can Make a Big Difference.* Boston MA: Back Bay Publishing.

Goldberg, E. (2005). *The Wisdom Paradox: How your Mind can Grow Stronger As Your Brain Grows Older.* New York: Gotham Books.

Kelley, D. IDEO's David Kelley on "Design Thinking." *Fast Company Magazine,* February 1, 2009.

Lawrence-Lightfoot, S. (2009). *The Third Chapter: Passion, Risk, and Adventure in the 25 Years After 50.* New York: Farrar, Straus and Giroux.

Lehrer, J. (2012). *Imagine: How Creativity Works.* New York: Houton Mifflin Harcourt Publishing Company.

Lehrer, J. "How to be Creative," in *The Wall Street Journal,* March 10, 2012.

Levitin, D. (2006). *This Is Your Brain On Music.* New York: Dutton Publishing.

Levitin, D. (2008). *The World in 6 Songs: How the Musical Brain Created Human Nature.* New York: Dutton Publishing.

Marcus, G. (2012). *Guitar Zero: The New Musician and the Science of Learning.* New York: Penguin Press.

Peacock, Molly (2010). *The Paper Garden: An Artist (Begins Her Life Work) At 72.* New York: Bloomsbury Press.

Ratey, J. (2008). *Spark: The Revolutionary New Science of Exercise and the Grain.* New York: Little, Brown & Company.

Sweeny, M. (2009). *Brain: The Complete Mind, How it Develops, How it Works and How to Keep It Sharp.* Washington, D.C.: National Geographic Society.

Index